Experiences and Explanations of ADHD

Experiences and Explanations of ADHD: An Ethnography of Adults Living with a Diagnosis presents research on the lived experiences of those diagnosed with attention deficit hyperactivity disorder (ADHD). Drawing on in-depth interviews with adults diagnosed with ADHD, the book provides an examination of how the diagnosis is understood, used, and acted upon by the people receiving the diagnosis.

The book delves into the phenomenology of ADHD and uncovers the experiences of a highly debated diagnosis from a first-person perspective. It further considers these experiences within the context of our time and culture and contributes to a discussion of how to understand human diversity and deviance in contemporary society. Studying both societal conditions behind the emergence of ADHD, questions concerning everyday life with ADHD, and interpretations of the diagnosis, the book offers an analysis of the intertwinement of experiences of suffering and diagnostic categories.

This book will appeal to academics, researchers, and postgraduate students in the fields of cultural psychology and medical anthropology, as well as those with an interest in the sociology of diagnoses.

Mikka Nielsen is a postdoctoral researcher at the Centre for Health Research in the Humanities, University of Copenhagen, Denmark.

Cultural Dynamics of Social Representation

The series is dedicated to bringing the scholarly reader new ways of representing human lives in the contemporary social sciences. It is a part of a new direction – cultural psychology – that has emerged at the intersection of developmental, dynamic and social psychologies, anthropology, education, and sociology. It aims to provide cutting-edge examinations of global social processes, which for every country are becoming increasingly multicultural; the world is becoming one "global village", with the corresponding need to know how different parts of that "village" function. Therefore, social sciences need new ways of considering how to study human lives in their globalizing contexts. The focus of this series is the social representation of people, communities, and – last but not least – the social sciences themselves.

Series Editor

Jaan Valsiner
Centre of Cultural Psychology, Aalborg University, Denmark

Books in this series

Culture and the Cognitive Science of Religion
James Cresswell

An Interdisciplinary Approach to the Human Mind (Open Access)
Subjectivity, Science and Experiences in Change
Line Joranger

Educational Dilemmas
A Cultural Psychological Perspective
Luca Tateo

Experiences and Explanations of ADHD
An Ethnography of Adults Living with a Diagnosis
Mikka Nielsen

For more information about this series, please visit: www.routledge.com/ Cultural-Dynamics-of-Social-Representation/book-series/CULTDYNAMIC

Experiences and Explanations of ADHD

An Ethnography of Adults Living with a Diagnosis

Mikka Nielsen

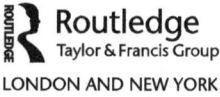
Routledge
Taylor & Francis Group

LONDON AND NEW YORK

First published 2020
by Routledge
2 Park Square, Milton Park, Abingdon, Oxon, OX14 4RN

and by Routledge
52 Vanderbilt Avenue, New York, NY 10017

Routledge is an imprint of the Taylor & Francis Group, an informa business

First issued in paperback 2021

British Library Cataloguing-in-Publication Data
A catalogue record for this book is available from the British Library

Library of Congress Cataloging-in-Publication Data
A catalog record has been requested for this book

ISBN: 978-1-138-30706-3 (hbk)
ISBN: 978-1-032-09014-6 (pbk)
ISBN: 978-1-315-14219-7 (ebk)

Typeset in Times New Roman by
Newgen Publishing UK

Contents

Series editor's introduction

Diagnoses in human lives: how social representations work

This book is about the power of invented labels – in psychiatric diagnoses – and about their constructive internalizations in human lives. Mikka Nielsen's coverage of these themes is thorough, deeply humanistic, and leads us all to further contemplation about how society functions through the persons who integrate the diagnoses into their own life courses as tools for personal development. It is here where social representations are brought into the domain of personal subjectivities – cutting across the person *versus* society dichotomy that the originator of the social representation theory, Serge Moscovici, intended all through his life.

The main link between the subjective and the societal worlds is the notion of *trust* – a topic that has been extensively covered in books published in this series (Markova & Gillespie, 2012) and in our *Advances in Cultural Psychology* series (Linell & Markova, 2014; Markova & Gillespie, 2007). There is a good reason for this recurrent interest. All human life depends on interpersonal trust – children need to trust parents, teachers, and policemen, their parents need to trust tax collectors and members of parliament, and some countries continue to retell everybody about their deep trust in deities – sometimes even on their bank notes. *Trust* is a hyper-generalized meaning field (Valsiner, 2019) and an ephemeral social representation that is very much in the core of human lives.

Yet trust is also subjectively fragile. It is one part of its relationship with its opposing systemic part – that of non-trust (Valsiner, 2018). This becomes particularly relevant if we start to look at the trust attributed to medical diagnostic labels or communicated via self-help books (Madsen, 2015). Most of Nielsen's eloquent coverage of the phenomena of cultural functions of diagnostic labels deals with this dialogue.

Personally, I find the trust in diagnoses – especially psychiatric diagnoses – weird. Growing up in Estonia under Soviet rule we learned from early on not to trust the claims made by various state institutions about their benevolent intentions towards individuals. This healthy distrust has served me well ever since. Going to a psychiatrist was represented back in Estonia as a shameful and potentially dangerous act. Which it was – a friend of mine who had naively sought consultation by psychiatrists for his teenage transition issues was later denied entrance to study psychology at the university. My apprehension had good reasons. Psychiatrists' services to the political establishments in various countries could be seen to give evidence for the need for distrust. Under deep belief in some ideological camouflage of brutal social power – such as communism in the former Soviet Union – diagnostic labels became widely used to take away basic human rights from individuals who elected to believe differently. Psychiatrists can easily be made into power tools in the regulation of any society – like in imperial Russia or the Soviet Union against deep religious believers (Windholz, 1985).

What Nielsen describes in this book is very different, as it pertains to the "happy country" of Denmark. It is strange how the journalistic attribution of the label "the happiest place in the world" easily becomes accepted by the ordinary populace – another example of the power of social representations. Denmark in the 2010s of course is very different from the Soviet Union of the 1930s and my native Estonia in the 1970s. It is a social welfare state based on the "Scandinavian model" of social contract relations where insiders in the societal system are given substantial privileges – supported by the high taxation rates – to make their lives affluent, and maybe even "happy". This leads to a situation where having a diagnosis can bring various benefits to the person. As a result having a diagnosis often becomes personally desired – like wearing branded clothing. This is a good example of the power of semiosis in value construction. Even after six years of experience in Scandinavia I still find such transformation of value a strange cultural condition not shared with most of the rest of the world. As a result – a by-product of the acceptance of the social contract of the welfare state – entertaining the diagnoses that are put on oneself becomes a *resource* in life-course development becomes understandable. Nielsen describes details of such phenomena in this book.

The widespread use of the attention deficit hyperactivity disorder (ADHD) diagnosis in our societies in recent decades and its personal and social implications constitute an interesting "natural laboratory" of societal becoming. Nielsen raises important issues that stem from her fieldwork. What happens if the person compensates enough for his or her difficulties to actually no longer meet the criteria for a diagnosis? When, if ever, is an ADHD diagnosis withdrawn? The whole issue of withdrawal of any psychiatric diagnosis – in contrast to somatic ones – is an issue needing further inquiry. I can be cured from syphilis, or pneumonia, or even cancer – the diagnosis is withdrawn after the success of antibiotics or radiation therapy. I do not get a negative stigma from becoming a "former cancer patient" – but would this be similar to becoming a "former schizophrenic"? How do societal sieves based on the collective affective social representations handle the organization of human life courses? Furthermore – does becoming a "former schizophrenic" eliminate the person's identity that had developed under the conditions of the diagnosis? Psychology has potentially much to offer to deal with these issues – that pertain to medical ethics and the role of healing efforts in all societies (Chaudhary, Anandalakshmy, & Valsiner, 2014; Joranger, 2018). There are more open questions in this book than there are answers. And this is good. Books that close human minds to new inquiries – the ones with fixed recipes for living – are the information noise that stops our minds from finding new solutions to perennial problems. Mikka Nielsen invites us all to open our minds – and I hope the readers will be ready for this intricate journey.

References

Chaudhary, N., Anandalakshmy, S., & Valsiner, J. (Eds.) (2014). *Cultural realities of being: Abstract ideas within everyday lives*. London: Routledge.

Joranger, L. (2018). *Subjectivity, science and experiences in change*. London: Routledge.

Linell, P., & Markova, I. (Eds.) (2014). *Dialogical perspectives on trust*. Charlotte, NC: Information Age Publishers.

Madsen, O.-J. (2015). *Optimizing the self: Social representations of self-help*. London: Routledge.

Markova, I., & Gillespie, A. (Eds.) (2007). *Trust: Dynamic and cultural perspectives*. Charlotte, NC: Information Age Publishers.

Markova, I., & Gillespie, A. (Eds.) (2012). *Trust and conflict: Representation, culture, and dialogue*. London: Routledge.

Valsiner, J. (2018). Civility of basic distrust: A cultural-psychological view on persons-in-society. In G. Marsico & J. Valsiner (Eds.), *Beyond the mind* (pp. 339–362). Charlotte, NC: Information Age Publishers.

Valsiner, J. (2019). *Hyper-generalization by the human mind: The role of sign hierarchies*. Hans-Kilian-Prize Lecture. Giessen, Germany: Psycho-Sozial Verlag.

Windholz, G. (1985). Psychiatric commitments of religious dissenters in Tsarist and Soviet Russia: Two case studies. *Psychiatry, 48*, 329–337.

Preface

This book evolved from my PhD project about ADHD and adults' experiences of receiving a diagnosis as a PhD fellow at the Department of Communication and Psychology at Aalborg University. The PhD project was part of a larger research project "Diagnostic Culture", funded by the Danish Council for Independent Research and carried out from 2013–2016.

The aim of the Diagnostic Culture research project was to contribute to current discussions about psychiatric diagnoses by investigating the high prevalence of psychiatric diagnoses, using depression and ADHD as representatives of the diagnostic expansion. Employing a three-angled strategy, the research project more specifically asked how adults experience the process of receiving a diagnosis of either ADHD or depression; how depression and ADHD are constituted in public discussions in popular media; and finally, how these diagnostic categories have emerged and developed historically.[1] The three perspectives each provide a crucial element in understanding how diagnoses spread throughout history and within societies and in gaining insight into personal experiences of living with a psychiatric diagnosis. Moreover, the perspectives combined allowed for the study of two apparent paradoxes: how diagnoses, on the one hand, are associated with shame and stigma, but, on the other hand, are often welcomed by the people receiving a diagnosis. Likewise, the perspectives support an analysis of how psychiatric diagnoses, on the one hand, are critiqued for their constructed quality, yet, on the other hand, have real-life effects on individuals' self-perceptions and opportunities in life.

The Diagnostic Culture research project was my academic base and initial entry into the field of ADHD. From this project, and in collaboration with the wonderful members of the research group, I developed and carried out my project about adults' experiences of ADHD. The ambition of the research project of combining macro- and micro-sociological and psychological perspectives, and to provide both a diagnosis of the culture and a cultural analysis of diagnoses (Brinkman et al., 2014, p. 692), was a great inspiration to my research. In other words, this book is an attempt to examine ADHD as a phenomenon, situated in the midst of personal experiences and cultural practices and perceptions of the human being.

Ethnographic fieldwork: examining experiences of ADHD

Since I started my ethnographic fieldwork on ADHD, I knew that ADHD was a controversial and contested diagnosis, often criticized for being a trending or bogus diagnosis, and I recognized that the complexity of ADHD was difficult to capture. In order to illustrate the complex character of the diagnosis, I wanted to include diverse accounts of ADHD. This book, therefore, is based on both historical and sociological analyses of ADHD as well as ethnographic data collected over a three-year period.

My initial encounter with ADHD, as it is managed in the clinical room, was facilitated through contact with helpful doctors at a clinic of general practitioners. The clinic opened the doors for me, allowed me to participate in consultations when their patients accepted it, and thereby established contact with some of their patients. This strategy enabled me to meet patients recently diagnosed and with very different experiences of being diagnosed. Besides recruiting participants from the clinic, I posted a request on an online forum for adults diagnosed with ADHD, asking for participants to the research project. The forum offered an open space for people to discuss ADHD-related subjects, and people recruited from this platform all chose to participate in a forum debating ADHD-related issues and to actively contact me. Hence, using this channel for recruitment gave access to people who could relate to the diagnosis of ADHD, who were searching for information about the diagnosis, and who would benefit from discussing the diagnosis with others. This second strategy therefore potentially precluded me from getting access to people diagnosed with ADHD who were less concerned with the diagnosis or maybe even opposed the diagnosis. In general, as with any research project, some limitations in regards to recruitment must be taken into account when reading and assessing the analyses. Considering that I lost contact with a number of participants during my fieldwork (due to their own private problems and struggles), the people who ended up participating in the project may represent some of the more resourceful people diagnosed with ADHD (even if they also had difficult periods during the period I came to know them).

My interlocutors were occupied within a wide range of professions, from working in sales, being a social and health care assistant, studying, working as a mechanic, as an IT technician, and being on a working-ability testing programme. They were aged between 26 and 45 and had all been diagnosed with

ADHD within the last five years. Without exception, they had experienced periods in life with symptoms of stress or depression and had been compelled to accept shorter or longer periods of sick leave. The diagnosis was often given after a period of stress and potentially sick leave from work, or it was given following the diagnosis of a child, or alternatively a combination of both. As an example, one of my interlocutors, Christian, told me how he had experienced periods of unhappiness and of not functioning well throughout his life. He remembered being bullied as a child, because he was different from the other children, and the feeling of not functioning well continued during adolescence. When he started studying, the pressure of administrating reading schedules and deadlines became too overwhelming. First, he was diagnosed with depression and was prescribed anti-depressants, but the bad periods kept returning and he unfortunately had to quit his studies. At that time, he was referred to a psychiatrist, who diagnosed him with ADHD. Like Christian, another of my interlocutors, Judith, remembers childhood feelings of being different. However, she was never in contact with the psychiatric system until her son was diagnosed with ADHD. As part of her son's diagnostic process, Judith started to do research on ADHD, and while reading about the diagnosis, she not only recognized her son but also herself in the diagnostic descriptions. Convinced she also had ADHD, she consulted a psychiatrist who subsequently diagnosed her with ADHD, just like her son.

Listening to stories of ADHD like Christian's and Judith's was a fundamental part of the research process for this book. The interviews generally focused on the person's life story, the diagnostic process, understandings of ADHD, what it meant to be diagnosed, everyday difficulties, and the effects of medication. I was invited into the homes of my interlocutors, and like Christian and Judith, they shared their life stories with me. They informed me about life with ADHD and they challenged me on my tentative ideas throughout the research process. The longitudinal ethnographic fieldwork made it possible for me to continuously develop new interests from the stories I was told, and share my initial analyses with the people I came in touch with. Just like I was examining life with ADHD, so were they exploring how to live with ADHD, and I was grateful for being included in their everyday reflections and observations. The participants in the study diagnosed with ADHD both challenge and agree with public discourses of ADHD, and being able to critically discuss different perspectives with my interlocutors was of great value. During the fieldwork I also came to learn that interviewing not only provided me with verbal reflections on life with ADHD, it also gave access to an embodied knowledge about ADHD. While seated in the interview setting, I witnessed the restlessness and the difficulty with concentration that I was verbally informed about, manifested in their way of speaking and being in the room. Confronted with these verbal, sensory, and bodily expressions of ADHD, I started to realize that understanding this disorder entailed an exploration of ADHD as more than a contested diagnosis that people interpret their difficulties through, but that ADHD is also a certain way of experiencing and being in the world.

As part of the ethnographic fieldwork, I participated in a variety of seminars and conferences for people diagnosed with ADHD, their relatives, and professionals working with ADHD. Together with observations from consultations with general practitioners and psychiatrists, as well as observations on online forums and blogs about ADHD, these observation studies offered a glimpse into spaces where ADHD is explained, negotiated, and managed. The observations enabled me to observe how ADHD is discussed and expressed in different social settings and they contribute to my research as background for understanding the context in which my interlocutors experience ADHD. From my observations in the clinical rooms, I saw how evaluation of dosages and changes in types of stimulants was a central theme. The conversations about medication were not only initiated by the doctor but also by the patient, and the observations gave me a small glimpse into the institutional and biomedical regime that the individual is included in when getting a diagnosis. Attending the seminars taught me about the official explanations of ADHD, ideas about coping with ADHD, and following the online forums and blogs I got an insight into the interests of people diagnosed with ADHD who use these forums for exchanging views and ideas. Moreover, these forums clearly illustrate how an ADHD diagnosis is both a category that the individual relates to and makes use of and a category to share with others diagnosed with ADHD within certain communities. Seminars as well as online discussions were well attended and the debates were vibrant with the participants exchanging ideas, experiences, and everyday tips.

All empirical data is collected in Denmark, a country known for being one of the most economically equal countries in the world and for its efficient welfare and health care systems. Consequently, concerns regarding insurance and coverage of medical expenses are not as central to my interlocutors, as they would probably be in, for example, an American context. A diagnosis, however, is still fundamental in Denmark in order to get access to resources and privileges such as sick leave from work, support for keeping the house, and of course medical treatment. Moreover, a diagnosis often brings about sympathy and legitimacy, just as it contributes to answering questions regarding identity and opportunities in life. My focus, therefore, is to chart some general developments behind the increase in ADHD diagnoses and to examine experiences of living with a diagnosis not only in Denmark but in Western society more generally. Since the increase in numbers of people diagnosed with ADHD in Denmark reflect a phenomenon that is spreading in most Western societies, the context of my study includes a variety of cultural, medical, and scientific tendencies and practices.

The names of my interlocutors and personal information have been changed in order to ensure anonymity.

Note

1 For further details see www.dc.aau.dk.

Reference

Brinkmann, S., Petersen, A, Kofod, E. H., & Birk, R. (2014). Diagnosekultur: Et Analytisk Perspektiv på Psykiatriske Diagnoser i Samtiden. *Tidsskrift for Norsk Psykologforening, 51*, 692–697.

Acknowledgements

I owe a great thanks to my interlocutors. You invited me into your homes and unreservedly shared your thoughts and life stories with me. I am truly grateful for your open-hearted, frank, and intelligent descriptions of both extraordinary, life-changing events, and of mundane, everyday activities and considerations. I hope I do justice to your stories with this book. I also want to thank the people at the medical practice *Sløjfen* who welcomed me at the clinic, let me participate in consultations, as well as put me in contact with potential interlocutors.

The importance of the Diagnostic Culture research group to the development of this book cannot be emphasized enough. Thanks to Svend Brinkmann, Anders Petersen, Mette Toft Rønberg, Ester Holte Kofod, and Rasmus Hoffmann Birk. My first initial analyses sprang from this research project, discussions within the group have guided my thinking, and a number of the sketches have been commented on and challenged by co-members. I am grateful for having been part of this group and I want to thank all of you for your constructive critique and for being the best colleagues one could ever wish for. I also want to thank Brady Wagoner who encouraged me to write this book.

Chapter 1

Introduction

When I first met Karen, one of the first things she said to me was, "I am hyper on my speech". Karen is 45 years old and was diagnosed with attention deficit hyperactivity disorder (ADHD) at 41. She agreed to be interviewed by me about her experience of living with ADHD, how symptoms of ADHD affect her everyday life, and what changes the diagnosis has brought about. Karen is an enthusiastic storyteller and she talked from the moment I switched on my digital recorder until the end of the interview, four hours later. From east to west, from one incident to another, and from yesterday's laughter and back to some of the darkest times in her life, Karen took me on a tour into her experiences of ADHD. Sometimes Karen lost track of her story and I needed to remind her where she started, but my interview questions were almost unnecessary as Karen honestly, figuratively, and humorously introduced me to her life with ADHD, a diagnosis she was given after numerous doctors' appointments and endless nights of speculations. Karen has struggled most of her life: in school, with her family, and at work. She has never kept a job for a long period of time, and has been in more relationships than most people. Karen's story whirled me into a life of disappointments when expectations from other people have not been met, when misunderstandings have ruined relations, and when family fights have torn her to pieces, but it also tells me about a life of managing to keep a family together against all odds and about a life where she is slowly beginning to find her footing.

I had just started my research project about ADHD a couple of months before I met Karen. And since ADHD was still an unexplored field for me, I asked her how she would explain what ADHD is to someone who does not know about the diagnosis. The picture she painted of ADHD as a clash of expectations and a life of constant challenges has stuck with me ever since:

> It is like approaching a candy vending machine, putting a dollar in it, and pressing "Daim" [chocolate bar]. And then you expect a Daim to snarf, but instead a boxing glove comes out, "boing", giving you a box on the ear.

To Karen, ADHD is about being different, about following a different logic, and about acting and speaking differently – and occasionally being knocked out for it. Like the boxing glove hitting her from out of nowhere. She once attended a seminar hosted by the Danish ADHD Association, where a presenter talked about speaking ADHD'ish, and she was thrilled to finally meet someone expressing so clearly what she had always believed: that she was somehow speaking another language. That she was simply always on the edge of how other people expressed themselves and experienced the world. Life with ADHD is a constant encounter with clashes and misunderstandings when different ways of thinking and acting collide, Karen tells me. Sometimes she manages to fit in and live up to the expectations of others. To behave according to other people's perception of what is appropriate. "I seem calm to you, right? But I can damn right promise you, I am not," she says, explaining how she twists her legs around the legs of the chair and keeps her arms crossed in front of her chest in order to keep herself restrained. "The whole body is locked." She knows that her restless movement, when she tries to ease her "craving for being hyper" is disturbing to others, and thus instead of moving her legs and fidgeting with her hands, she limits her cravings for movement by locking her body. This is her one of her strategies for adapting to other people's expectations. At other times, life hits her like a boxing glove. Karen has the courage of her own convictions, and sometimes she stands firm on her way of doing things differently, unaffected by the consequences. Then she is prepared for the boxing glove to hit. At other times, the boxing glove comes out of the blue.

Karen has always felt detached from her peers, but only after her daughter was diagnosed with ADHD and Karen started reading about the diagnosis, did she realize why. Karen was in the middle of a dramatic and evaluative time in life when she was diagnosed and she was struggling to hold her family together and keep custody of her children. She was in a legal fight with the father of her children and her relation to her mother was like an open wound. "I was tearing down and building up my life and I was reaching the point of being stuck, something needed to be done, but what the heck was I supposed to do?" After being rejected by several doctors who explained her difficulties as existential problems and left her by herself, Karen finally met with a psychiatrist who acknowledged her need for support and she got the ADHD diagnosis. Karen describes herself as someone who has always developed strategies in order to manage her difficulties, but at this time in life, she needed new strategies. The diagnosis became the help she was longing for and it facilitated a process of reflection that enabled her to understand herself in new ways. Medication following the diagnosis has been a great help that she says gives her "calmness and breaks for me to learn", and consultations (financed by herself) with a psychologist, who specializes in ADHD, help her "because he puts things into words". "A handicap," Karen tells me, "is when you do not understand, when the surroundings do not understand, and when no one is trying to explain". In that perspective, a diagnosis is the explanation that mitigates the handicap. It becomes the mediator between the clinical setting and life experiences and the translator, between the individual and his or her surroundings. It does not eliminate every experienced problem, but it helps you understand the clashes of everyday life and develop strategies for limiting conflicts and experiences of failure.

Karen's story is one of 13 life stories about ADHD I have listened to as part of my research on ADHD. All the 13 stories include unique lives and experiences in which ADHD plays a particular role. A small glimpse into Karen's story about ADHD illustrates elements of why and how some handle their problems through the help of a diagnosis and elements of what changes a diagnosis potentially brings about. Together with the additional 12 stories, Karen's story offers an insight into the complex lifeworld of restlessness, hopes, disappointments, and struggles connected to life with ADHD.

Aim of the book

This book is an examination of adult life with ADHD, embodied experiences of ADHD, the implications of being diagnosed with ADHD, and ways of relating to the diagnosis. Its ambition is to offer a nuanced insight into ADHD by presenting individual stories about ADHD and contextualizing these into a broader academic discussion about the increase in psychiatric diagnoses in general and the emergence of ADHD in particular. The book is concerned with questions such as, how can we understand experiences of racing thoughts, the head speeding, chaotic thinking, and bodily sensations of electricity running through the limbs, of thoughts jumping from subject to subject, and a continuous struggle for concentrating and sitting still? The American Psychiatric Association characterizes experiences like these as ADHD, which it categorizes as a neurodevelopmental disorder that comprises symptoms of inattention, hyperactivity, and impulsivity. In large numbers, people are diagnosed with ADHD and adults increasingly receive the diagnosis that was previously considered a diagnosis for children. But how do individuals experience getting an ADHD diagnosis as an adult and how is the diagnosis understood, used, and acted upon? Examining questions about the bodily experiences of what we call ADHD and the experiences of getting the diagnosis is the purpose of this book. It is an attempt to delve into the phenomenology of ADHD and unfold experiences of a highly debated diagnosis from a first-person perspective, and to understand these experiences within the context of our time, culture, and ways of understanding the human being. Studying both societal conditions behind the emergence of ADHD and questions concerning everyday life with ADHD and interpretations of the diagnosis, the book offers an analysis of the intertwinement of experiences of suffering and diagnostic categories, and contributes to a discussion of how to understand human diversity and deviance in contemporary society.

ADHD is a complex phenomenon and a relatively new psychiatric diagnosis. To understand what symptoms of ADHD feel like, why a growing number of people are diagnosed, why some people wish to be diagnosed, what explanatory force the diagnosis entails, and how it is received by the diagnosed, we need to address ADHD from multiple angles. The book will offer historical, sociological, psychiatric, and first-person perspectives on ADHD that collectively will create an assemblage of stories about the condition and hopefully contribute to an understanding of the complexity of ADHD and how to understand it as a disorder existing in time, place, and within social relations. My primary aim, however, is to present stories about life with ADHD, about experiences of struggling with a chaotic mind and a restless being, and about getting an ADHD diagnosis that describes these experiences. Research on adults' experiences of ADHD is limited, and considering the amount of psychiatric literature on psychopharmacological treatment, prevalence, and neurological aspects of ADHD, and of sociological literature on medicalization and the emergence of ADHD as a diagnostic category, the lack of research on how people experience living with ADHD is striking. We know very little about the effects of diagnosis and phenomenological aspects of ADHD as a way of experiencing and being in the world. I hope this book can go some way to remedy this lack and contribute to a hopefully emerging field of research on adults' experiences of ADHD. The aims of the book are therefore:

- To outline different explanations of the emergence of ADHD and the increasing numbers of people diagnosed with ADHD.
- To examine the impact of being diagnosed and how adults diagnosed with ADHD make use of the diagnosis when understanding themselves and their difficulties.
- To unfold an alternative perspective on how to understand experiences of ADHD in our time.

A diagnosis of our time

ADHD is, in many ways, a diagnosis of our time. Over the past decades, ADHD has been scrutinized, recognized, criticized, and treated in the Western part of the world, and the condition is linked to relevant questions concerning employability, insurance, and risk for accidental injury (Hinshaw & Scheffler, 2014, p. 132). From an anthropological point of view, focus on problems with attention interestingly reflects what we consider as deviant, inappropriate, and inadequate in our time – and maybe even how attention has become a scarce resource that is invested in and competed for (Kristensen, 2008). In an accelerating society with high performance criteria and with technologies constantly calling for our attention, an increase in the number of people diagnosed with ADHD requires an analysis of the dynamics between experienced symptoms of ADHD and societal developments.

The number of people being diagnosed with ADHD has increased rapidly since the diagnosis first entered the diagnostic manuals. We have also seen an increase in the number of prescriptions for drugs to treat ADHD. Teachers, psychologists, counsellors, and general practitioners refer people to psychiatric evaluations, but people also increasingly self-diagnose based on Internet tests, and actively visit their doctor in order to obtain an ADHD diagnosis (Conrad, 2007; Rafalovich, 2004). In my home country of Denmark, with a population of only approximately 5.6 million, the number of people prescribed drugs to treat ADHD has increased from 2,901 in 2002 to 35,554 in 2011, corresponding to a 1.125 per cent increase (Statens Serum Institut, 2012). In particular, adults represent a larger number in the statistics. While almost no adults were diagnosed with ADHD in 2001, 3,000 adults were registered as diagnosed with ADHD ten years later, and only within a three-year period, from the end of 2009 until the end of 2012, the number of adults receiving pharmaceutical treatment for ADHD has doubled (Statens Serum Institut, 2013). Newly revealed numbers of people in pharmaceutical treatment for ADHD in Denmark, however, indicate that the curve is flattening out (Sundhedsstyrelsen, 2015), and it will be interesting to see whether this reflects a new tendency. Nevertheless, a large group of people have been diagnosed with ADHD within the last couple of decades, and the diagnosis has not only spread within countries. The increase of people diagnosed with ADHD in Denmark echoes a general trend in Western countries, which some scholars describe as a "globalization of ADHD" (Conrad & Bergey, 2014) or even an "ADHD explosion" (Hinshaw & Scheffler, 2014). This research demonstrates that in countries such as Canada, the Netherlands, Germany, and Norway, rates of people diagnosed with ADHD have grown rapidly, despite varying diagnostic and treatment practices. These tendencies seem to be facilitated by several vehicles ranging from a transnational pharmaceutical industry, active advocacy groups, a competitive economic climate, to a general preoccupation with performance in educational and work settings.

Due to the increase in people diagnosed with ADHD within the last couple of decades, and to the migration of the diagnosis across countries, ADHD receives great public attention. As noted by sociologist Adam Rafalovich (2004), contemporary discussions about ADHD are represented by a plurality of both academic, clinical, pop-cultural, and journalistic views. The diagnosis is considered in TV shows, newspapers, and is heavily debated among professionals and laypeople. Famous actors, musicians, comedians, and business personalities have announced that they have been diagnosed with ADHD, and some even connect genius features in historical characters like Abraham Lincoln, Isaac Newton, and Socrates to ADHD (Schwarz, 2016). The diagnosis has become a category to identify with and that entails both positive and negative connotations. However, although some people succeed in transforming restlessness into accomplishments, most people diagnosed with ADHD experience severe difficulties and consequently seek medical advice (Hinshaw & Scheffler, 2014, p. 25). Treatment of ADHD is therefore also a hot topic in public discussions about ADHD and the dramatic rise in prescribed Ritalin and other central nervous stimulants has hit the popular media. In Denmark, headlines have brought massive attention to the diagnosis: "New Shock Numbers: 38,000 Are Taking ADHD Medication"[1] (Ritzau, 2013) and "Explosion: Adults on ADHD Medication Has Increased Twentyfold"[2] (Cuculiza & Weber, 2016). In 2014, the headline "Non-Treated ADHD Costs Nearly 3 Billion Kroner Each Year"[3] reached almost every Danish news media. The caption referenced a research project funded by a big independent research foundation, which estimated a massive reduced tax income due to, among other things, difficulties keeping a job and risks of committing crime among people with untreated ADHD (Rockwool Fonden, 2014). In 2013, the TV show *Denmark on Drugs*[4] critically portrayed the, according to the programme, alarming increase in the Danes' consumption of drugs prescribed for psychiatric conditions. A famous stand-up comedian diagnosed with ADHD hosted the programme and revealed that dramatic side effects from the medication led him to stop treatment. At around the same time, a whole range of other programmes aired on national television, such as *That's the Crazy Mind*,[5] *Mad or Normal?*[6] and *Dad, Mom and ADHD*,[7] all dealing with mental health issues and problems related to ADHD. These programmes took a different approach by challenging people's prejudices about mental illness and thereby reducing the stigmatization. The programmes aired parallel to the launch of a national campaign, "One of Us",[8] with the slogan "No More Doubt, Silence and Taboo About Mental Illness". The purpose of the campaign was to raise awareness about psychiatric disorders and to demonstrate that people with a psychiatric diagnosis are just like the rest of us. Whether the expression that people with a psychiatric diagnosis, are just like "us", i.e. as the people without a psychiatric diagnosis, is actually more of an excluding manoeuvre than the opposite, is worth considering (Brinkmann, 2016, p. 10). Nevertheless, the campaign, along with the myriad of TV programmes about mental health issues, demonstrates a tendency towards increased awareness about and a normalization of psychiatric diagnoses.

While critics of ADHD and stories about the increased number of drug prescriptions often attract headlines in the media, the voices of people diagnosed with ADHD hardly ever hit the headlines. Instead, people diagnosed with ADHD share their experiences, frustrations, and hopes in online forums, with their doctor, and among friends and family. Similarly, academic debates about ADHD within the social sciences are dominated by analyses focusing on the emergence of ADHD as a diagnostic category. Literature on experiences of ADHD is surprisingly limited and literature on adults' experiences of ADHD in particular is almost non-existent. The voices of the people being diagnosed are rarely examined, and there is a push for research on first-person perspectives on living with a diagnosis in general and with ADHD in particular (Comstock, 2011). From sociological research we know that diagnoses have multiple implications in institutional settings as well as on individuals' self-perception (Brinkmann, 2016; Conrad, 2007; Hacking, 2007; Jutel, 2011). Hence, diagnoses not only function as entries for treatment and resources, but also as carriers of explanations and self-understandings. Conrad (1976), Rafalovich (2004), and Singh (2007, 2011, 2013) contribute with valuable research on children's experiences of ADHD as well as their parents' conceptions of their children's diagnosis, but how ADHD in adults is experienced, interpreted, negotiated, and acted upon, remains almost unexplored and therefore deserves more public and academic attention.

An anthropological approach to ADHD

As a medical anthropologist, I understand individual suffering and illness experiences as social constituents, and I examine how available resources, languages, and treatments form the basis of individuals' perception of illness. Hence, what makes the study of experiences of ADHD interesting from an anthropological perspective is the complexity and the social dimensions of illness, and how individuals engage with and are shrouded in cultural understandings of illness. Even when studying experiences of ADHD, aspects of diagnostic practices and available treatment, conceptions of morality, and responsibility are entangled with the individual's experiences of ADHD.

Since the 1980s, there has been a request from the discipline of medical anthropology for research on illness experience and how illness is "lived through by the patient rather than conceptualized and defined by medical science" (Jackson, 1996, p. 6). The request reflects both a critique of the experience-distant worlds of a biomedical and social science discourse and a desire for an alternative to these perspectives (Willen & Seeman, 2012, p. 8). The purpose of this alternative focus on illness experiences, however, is not to disregard how medical categories affect experiences of illness. Rather, the ambition is to attend to the "peculiar qualities of the sting and throb of pain affecting a particular person – with a unique story, living in a certain community and historical period, and above all with fears, longings, aspirations" (Kleinman, Brodwin, Good, & Delvecchio, 1994, p. 2). Distinguishing analytically between illness and disease when describing respectively individual illness experiences and theoretical medical categories of pathology, anthropologist and psychiatrist Arthur Kleinman (1988) is widely recognized for addressing the difference in professional and personal interpretation of suffering, while at the same time acknowledging the intertwinement of the two. In the words of medical historian Charles Rosenberg (2002) we must acknowledge that we are "never illness or disease but, rather, always their sum in the world of day-to-day experience" (p. 258). The interest for medical anthropologists, therefore, is to point to the biological, cultural, and sociopolitical factors that underpin different illnesses as well as to the medical reasoning that shapes experiences of illness (Good, 1994; Lock & Nguyen, 2010). Kleinman (1988) states that, "[i]n every culture, illness, the response to it, individuals experiencing it and treating it, and the social institutions relating to it are all systematically interconnected" (p. 24), emphasizing how beliefs about sickness, behaviour exhibited by sick persons, expectations about treatment, and responses from practitioners are socially constituted. In this way, culture "fills the space between the immediate embodiment of sickness as physiological process and its mediated experience as human phenomenon" (p. 27).

Not only do medical anthropologists examine the intertwinement of illness and disease, research on illness experiences also points to the social aspect of experiences (Kleinman et al., 1994). Constructed in local "moral worlds", understood as the micro-context that mediates the relationship between societal and personal processes (Kleinman et al., 1994), experiences of suffering are only part subjective. They are also fundamentally intersubjective, as the experiencing individual continuously orients themselves in the world based on a sensibility to the local moral world. Universal occurrences such as, for example, death, disaffection, and disease, are experienced as particular forms of bereavement, pain, and suffering. Suffering not only affects the suffering individual, but it also has a profound effect on the lives of relatives and friends, who in turn shape the experiences of the sufferer. Therefore, to simply look at etiological mechanisms eschews what is essential in experience of suffering and the intertwined relationship between neurobiological and social psychological processes. Since experiences are always culturally constituted, so must mental illness be understood as engaging fundamental human processes, formed by culture, biology, and the psyche (Jenkins, 2015). Mental illness exists in families, in romantic relations, and at work, and manifests itself as a struggle, thwarting expectations and desires to navigate in these relations. In order to understand experiences of mental illness, we need to comprehend the social and cultural premises for experiences.

These anthropological analyses of illnesses and suffering teach us about the intersubjective aspect of experience, but they also encourage us as researchers to examine the local context of the experiencing individual. During my fieldwork, I came to learn that experiences of ADHD are intertwined with the desire to be a good parent, to be able to navigate in society, to keep a job, maintain friendships, and be socially accepted. Taking medication and experiencing a newfound calmness when reading bedtime stories for one's children render the quest for being a good parent possible, as I describe in Chapter 4. In Chapter 5, I explore how experiencing ADHD as both a way of being human and as an entity to distance from, illustrate how scientific and public explanations of ADHD form ways of understanding oneself. And Chapter 6 discusses how experiences of restlessness and having the feeling of being socially "out of sync" with people around you provoke the feeling of being different and misunderstood. Whether I examine bodily experiences of ADHD or experiences of getting and relating to the diagnosis, it is clear that experiences of ADHD are socially embedded. My interlocutors orient themselves in the world based on expectations from themselves and others and their experiences of ADHD are shaped by and situated within relations to others. Certain ways of being in the world and certain ways of understanding oneself are available within local contexts, and experiences of ADHD exist within these particular circumstances. In this book, it is my ambition to focus on my interlocutors' particular experiences, understanding these experiences in relation to social relations, family struggles, and cultural explanations of suffering, and expectations of being human, without understanding these experiences as simply products of social and cultural dynamics but rather in constant relation to them. Pointing to the increase in psychiatric diagnoses of different types of suffering and to laypeople's use of the diagnostic language in everyday conversations, I examine some of the many mechanisms that form our (Western) ways of understanding and experiencing suffering. I describe some of the mechanisms of how the diagnostic understanding of suffering has spread into individuals' vocabulary and self-interpretations and I examine individual experiences of ADHD, shaped by and acted upon within this diagnostic logic. By investigating cultural explanations for ADHD, moral responsibility, moral crafting of the self, and intersubjective and phenomenological aspects of ADHD, I chart different aspects of experiencing and being diagnosed with ADHD.

Clarifying concepts: ADHD as experience and diagnostic category

Throughout the book, I use the term ADHD to describe my interlocutors' experiences of what they portray as symptoms of ADHD, as well as when I refer to the diagnostic category. I will elaborate on the diagnostic manuals' definition of and the clinical criteria for diagnosing ADHD specifically in Chapter 3, but an initial explanation of my use of the term ADHD might provide some clarification.

Sometimes I refer to "what we call ADHD today" to underline the fact that ADHD is a contemporary term that defines and describes a specific set of symptoms at a specific time in history. I have no intention, however, of deconstructing the diagnosis, and I consider ADHD to be real in the same sense as anthropologist Emily Martin describes bipolar disorder as real: namely, that the reality of the disorder "lies in the cultural contexts that give particular meanings to its oscillations and multiplicities" (Martin, 2007, p. 29). Professionals, the public, and people experiencing the set of symptoms included in the diagnostic criteria all describe this phenomenon as ADHD, and they attribute certain characteristics to this description. Therefore, following the tradition in anthropology of using emic concepts, I use the term ADHD when I describe what my interlocutors are suffering from. Martin (2007) uses the phrase "living under the description" (p. 10) of a diagnosis in order to reflect that people are given a diagnosis and she calls attention to the fact that the diagnosis is only offering one description of a person. The phrase is useful to underline that ADHD is inscribed upon individuals based on certain criteria, which a phrase such as "people with ADHD" does not indicate. However, I prefer to use the phrase "people diagnosed with ADHD" when specifying that the individual is given a diagnosis in order to avoid what I perceive as an inferior position when talking about living *under* a description. From a stigmatization perspective, to be *diagnosed* with a condition could have the same connotations as above, but since diagnoses are no longer only put on individuals, but are often demanded from people and perceived as a resource, I find this phrase more neutral.

All the people I have interviewed were diagnosed with ADHD when I met them, which means they already relate to the diagnosis and interpret their experiences through the diagnostic descriptions in different ways. Therefore, to separate illness experiences and the diagnosis is complicated, if not impossible (a more detailed elaboration of the relation between illness experiences and the diagnosis will be dealt with in Chapters 4 and 5). I also examine ADHD as a certain way of being in the world and by that I recognize that the ADHD diagnosis covers a specific way of experiencing, struggling, and managing life (see Chapter 6). I believe that the people I have interviewed suffer from many of the same problems and that these problems should be acknowledged and addressed. Experiences of illness are distributed along a qualitatively defined continuum and it is not a question of either/or but rather to what degree people experience symptoms of a particular diagnosis (Hvas, 2015; Jenkins, 2015). Whether the ADHD diagnosis and the following treatment is the right solution for people experiencing symptoms related to ADHD are not the focus of this book, but I pragmatically recognize ADHD as a diagnosis that describes certain behaviour and sensations and that people relate to and interpret themselves through the diagnosis.

Structure of the book

The book is structured into five chapters, each presenting different stories of ADHD, and a final conclusion, which points to some recommendations for practice. While Chapters 2 and 3 outline current discussions within academia about ADHD as a diagnostic category, Chapters 4, 5, and 6 engage in these discussions by integrating ethnographic material from my fieldwork on ADHD.

In Chapter 2, I introduce different studies on examinations of deviant child behaviour, diverse explanations of the emergence of ADHD, and research on the medicalization of behaviour. These descriptions of ADHD represent traditions within psychiatry, sociology, history, and psychology, and illustrate how mental illness must be understood within its scholarly, social, and cultural context. Scholars remain divided over the legitimacy of ADHD and while some see ADHD as a genuine disorder with a long history, others consider the diagnosis as a form of social control. Therefore, the chapter describes some of the premises behind the current discussions about the status of psychiatric diagnoses and how ADHD became an official diagnostic category.

In Chapter 3, I list the diagnostic descriptions of and clinical guidelines for treating ADHD. The chapter also includes an introduction to relevant literature on what a diagnosis is, what role diagnoses are playing in contemporary health care, and how diagnoses "act" and are being acted upon by the people receiving a diagnosis. While some studies pragmatically outline the consequences of being diagnosed, others are more critical of what is conceived as an expansion of a diagnostic gaze and a diagnostic language in society. Moreover, the chapter introduces theories about the biologization of mental illness and the effect of neuroscientific knowledge entering into various academic disciplines. And finally, the chapter discusses how these theories potentially change our conception of the human being in general and of mental illness in particular.

Chapter 4 deals with experiences and implications of being diagnosed with ADHD and illustrates how a diagnosis offers a certain narrative, into which the individual's life trajectory is interpreted. The chapter examines the formative process of getting an ADHD diagnosis and how the diagnosis is welcomed with both relief and with ambivalence and concerns. Moreover, it is described how new everyday practices and routines are changed following the diagnosis, and how medical treatment transforms the individual's way of perceiving and being in the world. These processes of understanding and experimenting with opportunities offered by the diagnosis reflect how the diagnosis is part of a self-evaluative and self-constitutive project of becoming and striving to become a good parent, friend, and partner.

Chapter 5 is an examination of how people diagnosed with ADHD creatively make use of the diagnosis as well as the explanation of it when understanding themselves and their actions. The chapter presents two general positions: The first position involves an identification with ADHD as a way of being human and a specific way of managing (and failing to manage) life based on certain neurological structures in the brain. The second position involves processes of distancing from ADHD by separating the self from ADHD, transferring ADHD into an entity, explaining ADHD as caused by neurochemical impulses, and disclaiming behaviour connected to ADHD. Lastly it is discussed how a neurobiological explanation of ADHD potentially reduces comprehensions of how to live and cope with symptoms of ADHD.

Chapter 6 offers an alternative perspective on ADHD. Based on the assumption that people experiencing symptoms of ADHD have an impaired sense of time, ADHD is examined as a matter of a phenomenological difference in rhythm and a certain way of being in the world that is constantly out of sync. In situations of clashes between temporal orientations, a kind of desynchronization occurs. It is illustrated how certain practices, what is called "time work", is performed in order to establish a kind of resynchronization. The chapter emphasizes the intersubjective and intercorporeal aspects of ADHD and suggests that ADHD is not only an individual phenomenon, but rather symptoms of ADHD appear in relations, clashes, and interactions.

Chapter 7 concludes the study and outlines the arguments and contributions discussed, points to avenues for future research on experiences of ADHD, and offers recommendations for practice and ideas for reflections based on the analyses provided in the book.

Notes

1 In Danish: "Ny [*sic*] choktal: Nu får 38.000 ADHD-medicin".
2 In Danish: "Eksplosion: Voksne på ADHD-medicin tyvedoblet".
3 In Danish: "ADHD koster ubehandlet 3 mia. kroner om året".
4 In Danish: *Danmark på piller*.
5 In Danish: *Sådan er det skøre sind*.
6 In Danish: *Gal eller normal?*
7 In Danish: *Far, mor og ADHD*.
8 In Danish: *En af os*.

References

Brinkmann, S. (2016). *Diagnostic cultures: A cultural approach to the pathologization of modern life*. London: Routledge.
Comstock, E. J. (2011). The end of drugging children: Toward the genealogy of the ADHD subject. *Journal of the History of the Behavioral Sciences, 47*(1), 44–69.
Conrad, P. (1976). *Identifying hyperactive children: The medicalization of deviant behavior*. Lexington, MA: DC Heath & Company.
Conrad, P. (2007). *The medicalization of society: On the transformation of human conditions into treatable disorders*. Baltimore, MD: Johns Hopkins University Press.
Conrad, P., & Bergey, M. R. (2014). The impending globalization of ADHD: Notes on the expansion and growth of a medicalized disorder. *Social Science and Medicine, 122*, 31–43.
Cuculiza, M., & Weber, C. (2016, 22 February). Eksplosion: Voksne på ADHD-medicin tyvedoblet. Retrieved from www.mx.dk/nyheder/danmark/story/25635453.
Good, B. (1994). *Medicine, rationality, and experience: An anthropological perspective*. Cambridge, UK: Cambridge University Press.
Hacking, I. (2007). Kinds of people: Moving targets. *Proceedings of the British Academy, 151*, 285–318.
Hinshaw, S. P., & Scheffler, R. M. (2014). *The ADHD explosion: Myths, money, and today's push for performance*. New York, NY: Oxford University Press.
Hvas, L. (2015). Retten til at Være Rask i en Diagnosekultur. In S. Brinkmann & A. Petersen (Eds.), *Diagnoser: Perspektiver, Kritik og Diskussion* (pp. 319–340). Aarhus, Denmark: Klim.
Jackson, M. (1996). Introduction: Phenomenology, radical empiricism, and anthropological critique. In M. Jackson (Ed.), *Things as they are: New directions in phenomenological anthropology* (pp. 1–50). Bloomington: Indiana University Press.
Jenkins, J. H. (2015). *Extraordinary conditions: Culture and experience in mental health*. Oakland: University of California Press.
Jutel, A. (2011). *Putting a name to it*. Baltimore, MD: John Hopkins University Press.
Kleinman, A. (1988). *The illness narrative: Suffering, healing and the human condition*. New York, NY: Basic Books.
Kleinman, A., Brodwin, P. E., Good, B. J., & Delvecchio, M. J. (1994). Pain as human experience: An introduction. In M. J. Delvecchio, P. E. Brodwin, M. J Good, & A. Kleinman (Eds.), *Pain as human experience: An anthropological perspective* (pp. 169–197). Berkeley: University of California Press.

Kristensen, J. E. (2008). Opmærksomhed Ønskes!. *Asterisk*, *42*, 20–23.

Lock, M., & Nguyen, V. K. (2010). *An anthropology of biomedicine*. Chichester, UK: Wiley-Blackwell.

Martin, E. (2007). *Bipolar expeditions: Mania and depression in American culture*. Oxford: Princeton University Press.

Rafalovich, A. (2004). *Framing ADHD children: A critical examination of the history, discourse, and everyday experience of attention deficit/hyperactivity disorder*. Lanham, MD: Lexington Books.

Ritzau. (2013, 14 April). Ny choktal: Nu får 38.000 ADHD-medicin. Retrieved from http://politiken.dk/indland/ECE1944560/ny-choktal-nu-faar-38000-adhd-medicin.

Rockwool Fonden. (2014). *ADHD koster ubehandlet knap 3 mia. årligt*. København, Denmark: Rockwool Fonden.

Rosenberg, C. E. (2002). The tyranny of diagnosis: Specific entities and individual experience. *Milbank Quarterly*, *80*(2), 237–260.

Schwarz, A. (2016). *ADHD nation: The disorder. The drugs. The inside story*. London: Little, Brown Book Group.

Statens Serum Institut. (2012). *Salget af ADHD-medicin fra 2002–2012*. København, Denmark: Statens Serum Institut.

Statens Serum Institut. (2013). *Nu kommer de voksne også i ADHD behandling*. København, Denmark: Statens Serum Institut.

Sundhedsstyrelsen. (2015). *National klinisk retningslinje for udredning og behandling af ADHD hos voksne – med forstyrrelse af aktivitet og opmærksomhed samt opmærksomhedsforstyrrelse uden hyperaktivitet*. København, Denmark: Sundhedsstyrelsen.

Singh, I. (2007). Clinical implications of ethical concepts: Moral self-understandings in children taking methylphenidate for ADHD. *Clinical Child Psychology and Psychiatry*, *12*(2), 167–182.

Singh, I. (2011). A disorder of anger and aggression: Children's perspectives on attention deficit/hyperactivity disorder in the UK. *Social Science and Medicine*, *73*, 889–896.

Singh, I. (2013). Brain talk: Power and negotiation in children's discourse about self, brain and behavior. *Sociology of Health & Illness*, *35*(6), 813–827.

Willen S., & Seeman, D. (2012). Introduction: Experience and inquiétude. *Ethos*, *40*(1), 1–23.

Chapter 2

An old disorder or a recent product of medicalization?

Understandings of mental illness have changed throughout history – both in terms of what is considered deviant and the explanations used for understanding disorders. New psychiatric diagnoses are included in the diagnostic manuals while others are redefined or even excluded. The literature on ADHD covers very different portrayals of the disorder and demonstrates a field of complexity and controversies between different interpretations of how to understand ADHD. A central question during the past decades has been whether ADHD is biological or social in nature, and even if some researchers note that it is too simplistic to succumb to the idea that ADHD is either a social or biological phenomenon, the debate between the two perspectives continues. Scholars remain divided over the legitimacy of ADHD and while some scholars view ADHD as a genuine disorder with a long history, others consider the diagnosis as a form of social control. As noted by Mayes and Rafalovich (2007), explanations for the underlying causes behind ADHD have changed throughout history based on shifting cultural attitudes and medical developments and even today the various interpretations of ADHD demonstrate "that ADHD is far from being unified by an all-encompassing discourse" (Rafalovich, 2004, p. 7). This chapter introduces different perspectives that contribute to understanding ADHD as phenomenon, including relevant studies on developments in psychiatry and explanations of the emergence of ADHD. These descriptions of ADHD represent traditions within psychiatry, sociology, history, and psychology, and illustrate how mental illness must be understood within different scholarly, social, and cultural contexts. The chapter describes some of the premises behind the current discussions about the status of psychiatric diagnoses and how ADHD became an official diagnostic category.

A story of ADHD as an ever-present disorder

Behaviour connected to what we call ADHD today has been described and identified in children over the last couple of centuries, and books about

ADHD tell an almost identical story of how different physicians have observed symptoms of hyperactivity in children throughout the history of childhood behavioural disorders. In the following section, I will outline the most common descriptions of how the history of ADHD is told. It is not my intention to determine whether or not symptoms of ADHD have always existed, but rather to use this historical overview to illustrate how ADHD is commonly perceived as having emerged as a diagnostic category and how symptoms of what we call ADHD today have been treated throughout the last couple of centuries. Through changing medical discoveries as well as comprehensions and explanations of deviant behaviour, a review of the history of ADHD contributes to an understanding of how we have come to think about the diagnosis and the people diagnosed today – or what Edward Comstock (2011) calls the proliferation of the "ADHD subject". Moreover, the review illustrates the close-knit link between how we conceive of this type of behaviour and conceptions of how it should be treated.

The incapacity of necessary attention

In 1798 physician Alexander Crichton published three books based on his clinical observations of what was referred to at the time as "mental derangement", including a chapter entitled "On Attention and Its Diseases" (Lange, Reichl, Lange, Tucha, & Tucha, 2010). Crichton (1798/2008) expatiated on the nature of attention and the morbid alteration of attention, which he found in children as well as in adults, even if the condition seemed to diminish with age. From personal observations of patients, Crichton identified what he called an "incapacity of attending with a necessary degree of constancy to any one object" (p. 203) and based on these descriptions he was heralded as one of the first scientists to provide an account of "mental restlessness". The people mentioned in Crichton's study were easily distracted by extraneous stimuli, incapable of keeping attention, and felt a mental restlessness. Crichton describes the condition and its consequences in the following:

> People walking up and down the room, a slight noise in the same, the moving a table, the shutting a door suddenly, a slight excess of heat or of cold, too much light, or too little light, all destroy constant attention in such patients, inasmuch as it is easily excited by every impression. The barking of dogs, an ill-tuned organ, or the scolding of women, are sufficient to distract patients of this description to such a degree, as almost approaches to the nature of delirium. It gives them vertigo, and headache, and often excites such a degree of anger as borders on insanity.

When people are affected in this manner, which they very frequently are, they have a particular name for the state of their nerves, which is expressive enough of their feelings. They say they have the fidgets.

(p. 203)

In contrast to the predominant thinking of the time, Crichton took a medical and physiological approach to "mental derangement" issues and asserted that inattention was caused by an unnatural morbid sensibility of the nerves that a person was either born with or that was caused by an accidental disease. Hence, inattention was for the first time described in the literature as a pathological phenomenon – an understanding that has dominated in both medical spheres and the general public since then. However, as the previous quote shows, Crichton not only focuses on the individual pathology, but he also directs attention towards the environment and the influence of external factors on attention. The condition was therefore examined as a complex issue that needed to be coped with by helping the people in question recognize that some circumstances precluded them from concentrating and eventually thriving (Smith, 2012, p. 29).

Whether Crichton actually described what we today call ADHD is debatable and his research is only included in part of the literature about the history of ADHD. First, Crichton did not mention hyperactivity in his accounts, meaning that a comparison to ADHD can be criticized for being retrospectively strained (Smith, 2012, p. 29). Second, Crichton's reflections on inattention are difficult to ascertain today as they are based on unspecified personal experience (Barkley, 2008, p. 206). Nevertheless, Crichton made some interesting deliberations on the etiology of inattention disorders that now, more than 200 years later, are still relevant in contemporary understanding of ADHD.

Children suffering from immorality

While some consider Crichton to be the first to describe early symptoms of ADHD, others claim that the identification of hyperactivity, inattention, and impulsivity in children, and a conceptualization of the symptoms as a medical phenomenon, has its roots in the early years of the last century. Doctor George F. Still is widely acknowledged as the first paediatrician who described children with so-called abnormal incapacity for sustained attention and a distinctive "fidgetiness". Still was interested in childhood diseases and published and performed several lectures about his findings, including the most well-known series, "Some Abnormal Psychical Conditions in Children", from 1902. In these lectures, Still described his clinical observation of 20 deviant children who had all committed crimes or repeatedly transgressed moral boundaries and how he found that these children all had deficiencies in volitional inhibition. The children were easily distracted and unable to focus for a long time (Mayes & Rafalovich, 2007). From his studies, Still was stunned by how these children repeatedly maltreated and inflicted pain on other children without feeling regret or stole needless things without any efficient motive. It seemed that punishment did not have any deterrent effect, as the children could commit the same misdemeanour within a few hours after the punishment (Still, 1902/2006). While the children's behaviour could be interpreted as symptoms of "imbecilic" behaviour, as analyses of children's misbehaviour often concluded at the time, according to Still, this particular kind of behaviour was not caused by intellectual shortage. The differentiation between children suffering from "mental retardation" and the children from his observations was a central concern in his lecturers and he repeatedly emphasized that these children were not necessarily less intelligent than other children of the same age. Instead, Still concluded that the children were suffering from immorality or a "defect of moral control" (p. 130), defining moral control as "the control of action in conformity with the idea of the good of all" (p. 126). Hence, the children's lack of moral control was due to "the overpowering of one stimulus to activity – which in this connexion is the activity contrary to the good of all – by another stimulus which we might call the moral idea, the idea of the good of all" (p. 127). Still did not consider this lack of moral control as an individual shortcoming, but rather a biological defect caused by a failure in development (Mayes & Rafalovich, 2007). In a time influenced by evolutionary thinking and eugenics, Still was inspired by the contemporary currents and hypothesized that the moral ineptitude and failure in development was in accordance with the phenomenon of evolution. Following this evolutionary approach, moral control was regarded as the very highest product of mental evolution and a morbid limitation of moral control was therefore thought of as a developmental defect. Despite his insisting on biological and morbid causes for the children's condition, Still did not suggest medical treatment for the children but instead a careful training involving environmental accommodations since he claimed that "moral control can only exist where there is a cognitive relation to environment" (Still, 1902/ 2006, p. 127). This relation to the environment needed to be strengthened in order for the children to develop their moral consciousness and be able to act within moral conformity.

Still's focus on morality and the children's constant violation of moral codes – as a discrepancy between the child and the environment – is still relevant in discussions of ADHD, as I will show later in this chapter. Furthermore,

Still identified some characteristics of the inattentive children that we still recognize today: namely that there is an element of heredity to the specific behaviour, the inattentiveness becomes visible between the ages of 7 and 12, there is a marked overrepresentation of boys, and the children's memory tends to be affected in a negative way. However, even if Still is acknowledged by many scholars for publishing one of the first accounts of ADHD, others claim that Still's work is better understood within the field of moral hygiene and discourses of "imbecility" and "idiocy" of that time (Comstock, 2011; Rafalovich, 2004). His work contributed to a new medical discourse focusing on biology, but whether or not the children in his study suffered from what we would categorize today as ADHD, is still unclear.

Minimal brain damage and anti-school behaviour

Another leading expert on mental impairment, Alfred F. Tredgold, who conducted clinical observations of children with attention and concentration difficulties in the 1920s, also explained their behaviour as a moral developmental deficiency. Tredgold introduced the term "minimal brain damage" (MBD), and thereby followed Still's conviction that the children's difficulties did not stem from a character flaw or lack of discipline but rather from physiology (Mayes & Rafalovich, 2007). According to Tredgold, the children suffered from an organic abnormality on the higher levels of the brain, and he thus made a pioneering link between behaviour and neurological impulses. Tredgold and his medical research colleagues proposed many hypotheses as to what caused the impairment in the brain, including among other explanations, an epidemic of encephalitis lethargica in 1922. At the time, clinicians encountered children with symptoms of impulsiveness, hyperactivity, and irritability – similar symptoms to Still's observations – and therefore connected these symptoms to neurological damages from the epidemic of encephalitis lethargica. Tredgold raised essential awareness on the influence of brain damage on behavioural disturbances, though he did it in light of evolutionism. Shrouded in evolutionary thinking, he argued that the location of the individual's sense of morality in the brain was a product of recent evolution and therefore more susceptible to damage. Damage to this area of the brain was therefore considered to explain why the children' were afflicted by their "moral deficiencies".

Today, it is interesting to notice Tredgold's observations of the specific hyperactive and inattentive behaviour being revealed in the school setting. According to Tredgold, brain damage went undetected until the children were confronted with school demands. In school, their shortcomings were exposed, and the children started to exhibit so-called "anti-school behaviour" (Mayes

& Rafalovich, 2007, p. 439). The argument that symptoms of what we characterize as ADHD today stay unnoticed until children are confronted with school demands is widely acknowledged. Moreover, the linking of behaviour and neurological impulses in the brain still dominates thinking about ADHD, as I will show in Chapter 3.

A question of neurology: the rise of medical treatment

Psychiatrists following Still and Tredgold continued researching children's inattentive and transgressive behaviour. The cluster of symptoms, however, was not defined as a diagnostic category until 1957 when psychiatrist Maurice Laufer presented the diagnostic label "hyperkinetic impulse disorder" for children with a so-called "organic drivenness" (Mayes & Rafalovich, 2007, p. 442). Laufer was employed at the Bradley home, a neuropsychiatric hospital for neurologically impaired children, headed by psychiatrist Charles Bradley. The paediatricians at the home regarded the children's difficulties as a conflict in emotional development caused by anomalies in the structure of the central nervous system. In the early 1930s, a neurosurgical remedy in the form of a spinal tap was performed on some of the children as an experimental treatment, but the quite drastic surgical procedure turned out to cause severe headaches (Mayes & Rafalovich, 2007). In response to surgery Bradley therefore started clinical experiments in 1937 with the amphetamine Benzedrine on the so-called "problem children" showing restlessness, hyperactivity, and distractedness. From his experiments, Bradley was able to demonstrate that children receiving the drug showed a decrease in their symptoms: they were not running around but behaving quietly, they lowered their voices, they did not rush into offensive discussions in the same manner, and they generally exhibited more "subdued behavior" (Bradley, 1950, p. 24). When taking the drugs, the children increasingly adhered to social norms, it seemed. Another positive effect of Benzedrine was a "dramatic acceleration of their academic progress" (p. 25) and Bradley noticed that Benzedrine, as it eliminated unwanted behaviour, served as a kind of performance optimizing drug.

Whereas Bradley believed the drug only addressed the deviant behaviour and not the psychological subject or some underlying pathology, he recognized that Benzedrine was not able to change the children's character and the emotional conflict that caused the specific behaviour, but only the symptoms thereof (Comstock, 2011). The idea that drugs were able to treat the underlying pathology behind the symptoms developed later, when for example theoretical models about chemical imbalances in the brain gained academic and public interest (see Chapter 3). But with Bradley's experiments and research, drugs were suddenly not only used for curing diseases, but also for controlling specific behaviour. As Comstock (2011) notes, drugs facilitated "new possibilities of identity through the synthetic production of desirable behaviours" (p. 52). In many ways, Bradley's use of amphetamine to regulate and reduce children's mental disturbances foreshadows the employment of stimulants in treatment of children's behaviour. Believing that drugs were able to eradicate unwanted behaviour, the treatment potentially helped the children to "lead a different kind of *existence*" (p. 54, italics in original). A new link between drugs and the self emerged during these years – a relation that became essential in psychiatric practices and in the discipline's understanding and treatment of mental illnesses (p. 54).

The DSM era

After decades of doctors offering different interpretations of children's behaviour and misbehaviour, a more coherent and systematized approach to diagnosing children with problems of inattention was established. With the publication of the American Psychiatric Association's *Diagnostic and Statistical Manual of Mental Disorders* (DSM), used for categorizing and collecting statistical information about mental disorders, versions of what we call ADHD today was officially described and recognized.

The DSM is a collection of diagnostic categories, or as the manual puts it: "a classification of mental disorders with associated criteria designed to facilitate more reliable diagnoses of these disorders" (APA, 2013, p. xli). According to the DSM, it is intended to "serve as a practical, functional, and flexible guide for organizing information that can aid in the accurate diagnosis and treatment of mental disorders" (p. xli). Similarly, the manual "facilitate[s] an objective assessment of symptom presentations" (p. xli) and psychiatric disorders thereby gain medical legitimacy by being listed in the DSM. Although being primarily designed as a guide to clinical practice, the manual also serves a purpose outside the clinic, as it offers what is described as a "common language to communicate the essential characteristics of mental disorders" (p. xli). Therefore, professionals such as psychiatrists and psychologists working in mental health care but also other kinds of professionals such as social workers and legal specialists, are able to communicate in a common language with reference to the DSM. The manual is critiqued for being a "mix of social values, political compromise, scientific evidence and material for insurance forms" (Kutchins & Kirk, 1997, p. 11), but yet its authority prevails.

The DSM has been revised several times; each revision reflecting different understandings of human suffering and problems – or as Blaxter (1978) puts it: diagnostic categories may be considered as a "museum of past and present concepts of the nature of disease" (p. 11). While the first edition of the DSM did not leave much space for childhood disorders, the following versions of the DSM have included different versions of what we call ADHD today. By the 1960s, the term MBD was challenged and accused of being speculative, since no solid empirical data could validate if organic lesions in the brain were the actual cause of the behavioural pattern of children exhibiting poor attention and hyperactivity. Instead focus shifted to behaviourally defined syndromes based on observations of children. In the following, different versions of what is today called ADHD are listed (the diagnostic criteria for ADHD in the DSM-5 is more thoroughly outlined in Chapter 3).

- In 1968, the DSM-II coined the label "hyperkinetic reaction of childhood" and the concept of hyperactivity was incorporated in the official diagnostic classification manuals for the first time. Overactivity, restlessness, distractibility, and short attention span were described as core symptoms of the disorder, and the two distinguished features, hyperactivity and inattention, were clustered together, just as they are in today's diagnosis of ADHD.
- In 1980, the DSM-III renamed the disorder "attention deficit disorder (ADD) (with or without hyperactivity)" and emphasis changed from hyperactivity towards inattention. Inattention was considered a more significant feature than hyperactivity, and in addition, inattention showed the best response to stimulant treatment. Hyperactivity, though, was included in the name of the diagnosis in a revised version of the DSM-III, and "attention deficit hyperactivity disorder" (ADHD) was introduced in the DSM-III-R in 1987.
- The DSM-IV, published in 1994, continued with the term ADHD, divided into three specific subtypes (predominantly inattentive, predominantly hyperactive-impulsive, and combined). This edition tentatively expanded the definition of ADHD by including examples of workplace difficulties in the diagnostic descriptions and thereby proposing that ADHD was not exclusively a child disorder.
- However, not until the release of DSM-5 did the manual explicitly present a diagnostic description for adults in order to "facilitate application across the life span" (APA, 2013, p. 809). While symptoms of hyperactivity often become less obvious in adolescence and adulthood, the DSM states that difficulties with restlessness, inattention, and impulsivity persist and that a "substantial proportion of children with ADHD remain relatively impaired into adulthood" (p. 62). Hence, when introducing the DSM-5, diagnosing adults was officially authorized.

A one-sided story of ADHD?

The above history of ADHD tells a story of the pathologization of certain patterns of behaviour, and the development of a diagnosis based on perceptions of illness and treatment available at the time. It also tells a story of a given period, when behaviour that was not previously treated within the medical field was suddenly considered as pathological and requiring treatment. In spite of changing medical perspectives, similarities between the different categorizations of behaviour and explanations are noticeable: The question of whether the disorder is caused by brain mechanisms has persisted, and even if the MBD hypothesis was abandoned and focus shifted to observations of behavioural patterns, the assumption that deviant behaviour is caused by a brain dysfunction prevails in different versions among researchers and clinicians throughout the history of ADHD (Timimi & Leo, 2009). Further, the tradition of prescribing stimulants to children with behavioural problems started years before the ADHD diagnosis was established, even if it did not become regular practice before Ritalin was introduced in the 1960s (Smith, 2012). The idea that the children's problematic behaviour is caused by a dysfunction in the brain can be traced back to both Bradley and Still, and today's theories about hyperactivity and inattention seem to follow some of the same ideas about the dynamics between behaviour, brain mechanisms, and medical treatment: ADHD is a neurobiological disorder, because drugs are the most effective treatment, and drugs not only treat symptoms, but address the brain mechanisms that produce the symptoms (Comstock, 2011).

Some researchers critique the story of ADHD for being too selective, putting too much emphasis on specific types of behaviour, and leaving out factors that might tell a different story of the children in question in order to legitimize current conceptions of ADHD. According to historian Matthew Smith (2012), the stories of hyperactivity follow a similar pattern in the description of hyperactivity because they share the same purpose of depicting hyperactivity as an ever-present neurological condition that has little to do with the social environment. A certain story about ADHD is told in order to verify that what we call ADHD today has always existed, and to reject the position that ADHD as a diagnosis is a product of social and cultural conceptions of what is considered deviant. Moreover, Smith (2012) claims that the history matches the idea of medicine as progressive and ever improving. Instead, Smith (2012) advocates for a more nuanced historical analysis that contributes to the discussion of whether what we call ADHD today has always existed as problematic behaviour or if the diagnosis is a product of our time and specific social arenas and medical regimen. Smith's historical analysis of ADHD is elaborated in the following section among other analyses of why the number of ADHD diagnoses has increased over the years.

A critical explanation of ADHD

Chris Mercogliano (2009) writes that the world's struggling children diagnosed with various psychiatric diagnoses are like "canaries in a coal mine". This statement reflects a critical approach to ADHD that interprets children's behaviour and suffering as reactions to distress and indications of a polluted environment. Theories about social pathologies point to similar conclusions when understanding the increase in people experiencing certain kinds of suffering and receiving certain diagnoses. Common to these perspectives is the conception of problems of health and well-being as related to changes of social structures and possibly crises in the civilization as a whole (Keohane & Petersen, 2013).

As described above, the history of ADHD is generally portrayed in one of two ways: one is the story of how hyperactivity has been identified in children throughout the last couple of centuries but treated and understood within the changing medical profession; the other is the critical story of ADHD as emerging in a specific context in which political, environmental, and social factors have created conditions that either produce certain behaviour or under which certain behaviour becomes the centre of professional attention. In this section, I present some of the critical literature dealing with psychiatric diagnoses, diagnostic practices, pharmaceutical treatment, and medicalization of behaviour, which link the emergence of ADHD to societal and cultural changes.

Medicalization of society

One of the most influential and significant positions in theories about the emergence of ADHD is the argument that ADHD is a product of the medicalization of behaviour. Researchers suggest that the growth of medical jurisdiction is among the most influential transformations during the past decades in the Western world (Clarke, Shim, Mamo, Fosket, & Fishman, 2013, p. 161). Diagnoses increasingly demarcate what is acceptable and what is considered pathological, and behaviours and emotions that were once defined as immoral, sinful, or criminal, are now being diagnosed as medical problems and thereby transferred "from badness to sickness" (Conrad, 2007, p. 6). But why is the number of problems defined as medical problems growing? Why are, for example, hyperactivity and inattention defined as symptoms of a diagnosis and not simply perceived as bad behaviour? In order to understand and critically investigate the development of various phenomena being gradually understood and managed within a medical domain, sociologist Peter Conrad (2007) asks: Is there an epidemic of medical problems? Is the medical practice better at identifying and treating already existing problems? Or is a whole range of life's problems being diagnosed and subjected to medical treatment despite the dubious evidence of their medical nature? To answer the questions, Conrad claims, one must understand what medicalization implies.

Framed by Irving Zola (1972), medicalization as a concept describes the extension of medical authority and practice into increasingly broader areas in life. In theory, medicalization not only refers to problems whose medical status is questioned (such as the menopause and alcoholism), but also problems more generally accepted as rightfully treated within the medical professions (as for example epilepsy) (Conrad, 2007, p. 5). In practice, however, discussions about medicalization often take a critical stance, examining existential phenomena now being the subject of medicalization. Research on, for example, the medicalization of grief (Kofod, 2017) or ageing (Oxlund & Whyte, 2014) illustrates how medicalization potentially narrows the range of what is considered acceptable and diminishes our tolerance for and appreciation of the diversity of human life. The main problem with medicalization, therefore, is its transformation of human differences, struggles, and sorrows into pathologies. Further, medicalization is critiqued for locating the source of the problem in the individual rather than in his or her social environment and thereby calling for individual medical interventions rather than collective or social solutions. Conrad (2007) argues that the individualization of social problems obscures the social forces that influence our mental health, that it depoliticizes deviant behaviour by understanding behaviour only within a clinical rather than social and political frame, and by expanding the medical jurisdiction, medicalization increases social control over human behaviour and emotions.

Medicalization must be understood within its social and cultural context, and social factors such as the decline of religion, increased faith in science, the prestige of the medical profession, and penchant for technology to solve our problems all provide opportunities for medicalization to occur (Conrad, 2007, p. 8). Similarly, several drivers for medicalization can be identified, and especially patient organizations and the pharmaceutical industry have played significant roles, advocating for the medicalization of specific phenomena and promoting specific diagnoses. The two groups therefore mutually support each other, as both have an interest in medicalizing certain conditions for either the benefit of legitimization and access to resources or in order to profit from selling drugs. As an example, Conrad (2007) points to the American advocacy group CHADD (Children and Adults with Attention Deficit Hyperactivity Disorder), as a strong supporter for diagnosing ADHD and for treating the disorder with pharmaceuticals. CHADD has grown significantly over the past decades, owing much of its growth to the increase in adults diagnosed with ADHD (Conrad & Potter, 2000). But the success of the organization may also be due to the fact that CHADD is supported financially by the pharmaceutical industry, and it is no secret that the organization receives support from Novartis, the manufacturer of Ritalin (Conrad, 2007, p. 55). In the following section, the different drivers behind the medicalization of ADHD will be elaborated further.

Social, political, and cultural factors behind the emergence of ADHD

In his book *Hyperactivity: The Controversial History of ADHD*, Smith (2012) offers a historical account of hyperactivity and management of hyperactive behaviour. His research reveals how complex factors have come to shape our understanding of ADHD and the treatment thereof and why the increase in ADHD diagnoses happened during the post-war period. According to Smith, the rivalry between the United States and the Soviet Union, and the political climate following it, produced circumstances for ADHD to emerge. At the time, the workforce was to outperform other countries' scientific developments in a globalized world, and the disappearance of unskilled work required a technologically sophisticated workforce. Fearing that the Americans were losing "the brain race" against their rivals, new initiatives needed to be taken in order to improve the educational performance of the American population (p. 54). Any obstacle that interfered with the goals of educational achievement was considered threatening to the overall aim of winning the race against the Soviet Union, and politicians, educators, and researchers started analysing where to deploy resources. The answer was the children. The post-war period had experienced a baby boom and overloaded classrooms together with a shortage of good teachers creating what Smith refers to as a crisis in education. To meet this challenge, new educational strategies were developed. Education became the battlefield where the race was to be won and the relatively newly established reform pedagogy was replaced by a stricter pedagogy that required great discipline (p. 60). Moreover, the school counselor entered the classroom in order to help the teacher identify children who were struggling academically and disturbing the lessons and subsequently referring the children to a psychiatrist for diagnosis and treatment. Counsellors became the mediator between the educational and the medical sphere, recognizing and handling problematic behaviour. These factors collectively created an educational milieu where hyperactivity, impulsivity, and inattention became associated with academic underachievement and intellectual shortcomings. Children's behaviour became an important focus area, and with the increasing use of pharmaceutical drugs, the answer was obvious. The role of Ritalin, which Smith also points to in his analysis of the emergence of ADHD, will be dealt with in the following section.

Another critic of perspectives underestimating the social and cultural aspects of ADHD is psychiatrist Sami Timimi. Based on a review of critical literature on ADHD, Timimi (2009) posits two possible explanations for the increase in ADHD diagnoses: either there has been a real increase in ADHD-type behaviour, which has led to greater scrutiny and concern about the behaviour; or there is no real increase in ADHD-type behaviour, but rather we have come to think about and deal with children's behaviour differently. While both explanations seem reasonable, an interaction between the two, Timimi proposes, might give a clearer picture of what causes the increase in ADHD diagnoses. Changes in our cultural and environmental contexts produce an increase in ADHD-type behaviours, just as these changes in behaviour transform our perceptions of childhood behaviour, which in turn alter our common cultural practices around children.

First, environmental factors play a crucial role. Like Smith (2012), Timimi (2009) points to changes in the educational system, but emphasizes new teaching methods focusing on self-regulation and the highly stimulating environment in the classroom as key components for why children who have problems with attention struggle in school. Standard tests are introduced in class and energetic activities such as music and gym have been set aside, resulting in increased pressure on children's ability to concentrate on academic tasks (p. 139).[1] From this point of view, it is no surprise that children with difficulties related to attention and self-regulation are increasingly challenged in school. Moreover, there has been a so-called "moral panic" about boys underperforming in school, and whether or not boys' underachievement is a consequence of what some refer to as a "feminization" of the school that favours girls' behaviour – there is a noticeable gender gap in ADHD diagnoses (p. 150). Similarly, Rosenfeld and Faircloth (2006) describe what they call the "medicalization of boyhood" (p. 134) when explaining why boys comprise the majority of children diagnosed with ADHD.

Second, Timimi (2009) points to changes in how we think of children's behaviour and the role of parenting as a factor in the ADHD epidemic. As the national state has become continuously more interventionist in family life and parenting skills have become subject to surveillance, parents are more aware of their children's behaviour and tend to leave guidance of the children to the expertise of professionals, thereby delegating authority from parents to professionals in the upbringing of children (p. 140). Moreover, so-called "mother-blaming discourse", accusing failed motherhood for children's deficiencies, might also explain why mothers have actively demanded psychiatric diagnoses for their children, thereby transferring the cause from parenting skills to neurobiological explanations (p. 148). Generally, patients have become more engaged in the diagnostic process, as Conrad (2007) similarly claims, and parents increasingly play a role in the demand for a diagnosis.

Lastly, Timimi (2009) directs focus towards psychiatry and the pharmaceutical industry. According to Timimi, the number of psychiatric consultants in the UK has more than doubled in the past two decades and the increase in prescriptions of drugs to psychiatric patients corresponds with these numbers (p. 149). The pharmaceutical industry supports both patient activist groups and doctors' seminars at popular vacation sites, and Timimi argues that the role of the industry in the emergence of new diagnoses should not be underestimated. Furthermore, the search for quick-fix solutions in the form of diagnoses and pharmaceutical treatment reflects a general societal attraction to technological advances that apparently make life easier, and in that respect, drug treatment fits in perfectly with our craving for efficiency and accuracy (p. 151). Family therapist Marilyn Wedge (2015) presents a similar analysis, criticizing American psychiatrists for overdiagnosing and overmedicating children and drawing attention to France, where children are not equally diagnosed with attention disorders. According to Wedge, alternative guidelines for diagnosing together with strict parenting strategies explain "why French kids don't have ADHD", and her analysis points to how culture within both family structures and cultural attitudes towards medicine foster different circumstances for the increase in ADHD diagnoses.

Ritalin on the market

Throughout the critical literature about ADHD, Ritalin is described as a central factor behind the emergence of ADHD. Conrad (1976) even proposes that a cynical reading of the history of medicalization might be that "the label was invented to facilitate the use of a particular social control mechanism, in this case psychoactive drugs" (p. 15). Similarly, science journalist Robert Whitaker (2010) accuses the pharmaceutical company that produces Ritalin of misguiding their consumers when telling them that children with ADHD are suffering from low dopamine levels. The reason parents were told this story, Whitaker argues, is because Ritalin stirs neurons to release extra dopamine, and the company therefore had great interest in promoting the theory of ADHD as a consequence of low dopamine levels. Whitaker states that by identifying the mechanisms of a particular drug, the company transformed research about the effects of a drug into a theory of impairment.

Notwithstanding the level of cynicism, researchers point to the fact that Ritalin played a crucial role in the rise of the neurobiological explanation for hyperactivity. From the 1960s tests of the effectiveness of stimulant medication in hyperactive children (Comstock, 2011; Smith, 2012), to later advertisements for Ritalin, the neurobiological explanation subdued more psychological approaches. Because the drug promoted ADHD as a neuro-logical problem and not an issue of improper parenting or unhealthy envir-onments, parents and others involved in children's development welcomed the drug. Parents got a legitimate explanation for their children's behaviour, doctors got a concrete tool for treatment, and Ritalin thereby had the ability to generate a positive clinical encounter between patient, parent, and psych-iatrist (Smith, 2012).

Smith (2012) describes how Ritalin was first marked for different conditions such as obesity, narcolepsy, and depression, but its real success started when it was introduced as treatment for ADHD (p. 107). The company manufac-turing Ritalin marketed the drug heavily in films and guidebook publications for parents, and they even organized meetings for parents and teachers about hyperactivity (p. 116). The advertisements were not only directed at doctors, they also spoke to parents when infusing hope for getting happier and much calmer children.[2] An advertisement from a medical journal in the 1970s illustrates Smith's point: On one side of a page is an angry boy, playing with a wooden toy, which he has torn apart. With teeth clenched and eyes closed, the boy is pictured as unhappy, and the image is blurred as if the camera could not keep up with his movements. On the other side of the page, the child is much calmer, reading a book, and looking relaxed and quiet. Above the first picture, a caption states "how children with minimal brain dysfunction may be 'aggressive, destructive, easily frustrated' and 'can't concentrate'" (p. 101), while the second picture similarly has a caption declaring "how 'it may be that stimulants act on higher (cortical) centres of the brain and thereby 'stimulate' greater conscious awareness'" (p. 101).

Researchers in neuroanatomy and social work respectively, Leo and Lacasse (2009) also point to the link between the introduction of Ritalin and especially the advertising of the drug and the dramatic rise in the number of children diagnosed with ADHD. Leo and Lacasse (2009) highlighted the webpage ritalinla.com, hosted by a pharmaceutical company, which stated in 2008: "Studies show that the brains of children with ADHD may function differently than those of other children. These children may have an imbalance of chemicals in the brain that help to regulate behaviour" (p. 291). Another text informs us that: "While the specific cause has not been confirmed, brain imaging research using a technique called magnetic reson-ance imaging (MRI) has shown that differences exist between the brains of children with and without ADHD" (p. 289).[3] Leo and Lacasse (2009) note that radiological images of the brain have been used for marketing ADHD medications and that the consumers interpret the images as documenting a definable and visible neuropathological abnormality. The neuroimaging studies, however, are indefinite and just like the theory of altered biochemistry of the brain is both complex and contested, parents and other recipients of the advertisements are not necessarily aware of the scientific reservations of the research. While the medical literature shows conflicting results and is based on a continuous questioning of its results, the advertisements portray the research in a simplistic way that leaves the consumer to think that evidence for the biological aspects of ADHD are unambiguous and clear (p. 308). Proponents of these kinds of advertisements directed at the consumers might propose that the advertisements increase disease awareness and therefore raise general public health and, according to Leo and Lacasse (2009), patients actually increasingly bring their concerns about potential symptoms to the doctor after seeing these advertisements (p. 287). The result of more people searching for answers to their experienced problems within a medical context is, thus, that more people are getting the available answers within this context.

As this brief review shows, advertisements and marketing campaigns promised parents, teachers, and children relief from some of their most dominant problems at home and in the classroom, infusing them with hope for a better future. In many ways, however, as Smith (2012) puts it:

> Ritalin "worked" as a treatment for hyperactivity to the extent that it reduced the symptoms of 80 per cent of the hyperactive children who took it, but this is not the same thing as saying that it helped those children.
>
> (p. 125)

Clinical evidence as well as anecdotal stories point to the potential of Ritalin to help children struggling with inattention and hyperactivity. Nevertheless, whether or not drugs are the best solution is debatable, and questions of (long- and short-term) side effects, on the one hand, and the risk of overlooking social issues as the possible cause behind the child's behaviour, on the other hand, are still important factors to consider.

Diagnosing adults with ADHD

While ADHD was initially only a diagnosis for children, adults are now increasingly diagnosed as well. In 2002, Strattera became the first drug specifically approved and promoted for treating ADHD in adults, and as mentioned at the beginning of this chapter, DSM-5 explicitly included adults in the diagnostic descriptions. But how did ADHD, which for years was deemed a disorder of childhood, become a diagnostic category that also includes adults? What happens with psychiatric diagnoses over time, taking their fluid and arbitrary status into consideration? First of all, studies have revealed that symptoms persist into adulthood for some individuals diagnosed with ADHD as a child (Conrad, 2007, p. 50). But the notion of adult ADHD not only stems from this natural development, when diagnoses follow the individual into adulthood; other mechanisms also account for changes in both public and professional conceptions of who can be diagnosed with ADHD. In order to describe some of these mechanisms, Conrad (2007) has coined the concept of a "diagnostic expansion". Medicalization involves an elasticity, meaning that medical categories both expand and contract as new criteria are either integrated into or excluded from the diagnostic categories, as is demonstrated in the descriptions of ADHD in the DSM. The concept of diagnostic expansion describes the process of how "once a diagnosis is established, its definition, threshold, or boundaries can be expanded to include new or related problems or to incorporate additional populations beyond what were designated in the original diagnostic formulation" (Conrad, 2007, p. 47). Hence, the identification of ADHD in adulthood is a product of including new problems into a diagnostic category, and while childhood ADHD was a product of the medicalization of behaviour, Conrad (2007) claims that adult ADHD is a consequence of the medicalization of underperformance (p. 64). Adults diagnosed with ADHD often experience themselves as underperforming and not being able to live up to society's demands, and the diagnosis thus provides a medical explanation for their underperformance (p. 65).

In parallel to the diagnostic expansion of the medical category as an explanation of adults increasingly being diagnosed with ADHD, other social and commercial drivers are at play. A combination of media portrayals of ADHD, popular books about adult ADHD, as well as lay organizations and the pharmaceutical industry's advocacy for adult ADHD contribute to the proliferation of adults being diagnosed with ADHD. In the 1990s, books about ADHD in adulthood reached out to a big audience. In 1993, *You Mean I'm Not Lazy, Stupid, or Crazy?! A Self-Help Book for Adults with Attention Deficit Disorder*, by Kate Kelly and Peggy Ramundo, described how an ADHD diagnosis could bring a shift in responsibility among adults. The following year, Thom Hartmann (1994) published his book *Attention Deficit Disorder: A Different Perception*, in which he, within a sociobiological framework, associates ADHD with an evolutionary adaptation to the environment and links ADHD to the quality of prehistorical hunting skills. That same year, Edward Hallowell and John Ratey's book *Driven to Distraction* (1994) became a bestseller. The two authors draw on their own experiences of living with ADD and promise their readers that life with ADD can be successful. They write:

> The best way to think of ADD is not as a mental disorder but as a collection of traits and tendencies that define a way of being in the world. There is some positive to it and some negative, some glory and some pain. If the negative becomes disabling, then this way of being in the world can become a disorder. The point of diagnosis and treatment is to transform the disorder into an asset.
>
> (Hallowell & Ratey, 2005, p. xxxii)

The same year, 1994, the cover of *Time* magazine asked: "Disorganized? Distracted? Discombobulated? Doctors say you might have attention deficit disorder. It's not just kids who have it" (Conrad, 2007, p. 55). Simultaneously, the two actors promoting medicalization of ADHD in childhood, CHADD and the pharmaceutical industry, also advocated for ADHD in adults to be recognized. CHADD organized several conferences about adult ADHD, and the pharmaceutical company that produces Ritalin redefined ADHD as a lifetime disorder, drawing on arguments about ADHD as a genetic disorder. However, the massive promotion of ADHD was not without criticism and the following years books such as *Talking Back to Ritalin* (Breggin, 1998) and *Ritalin Nation* (DeGrandpre, 1999) critiqued the proliferation of ADHD and Ritalin use. Nevertheless, the attention in popular media towards ADHD led to a new trend of self-diagnosing among adults, who, after reading and hearing about the benefits of the diagnosis, increasingly demanded an ADHD diagnosis and thereby contributed to fueling the social engine of medicalization. While children were primarily referred to a psychiatrist by parents or teachers, adults had already self-diagnosed before meeting with a physician (Conrad, 1976; Rafalovich, 2004).

Conrad's (2007) analysis shows how the diagnosis is embraced and promoted by the people who receive it and how the widespread acceptance of diagnoses stimulates a diagnostic expansion. Self-diagnosis and self-referral are integral features behind the emergence of adult ADHD, and individuals' identification with and diagnosis-seeking behaviour might be one of the biggest changes in ADHD history (Conrad & Potter, 2000, p. 570). Laypeople's promotion of diagnosis and the widespread practices of self-diagnosing challenges some of the premises of labelling theories. The proliferation of diagnoses is therefore not only a consequence of the pharmaceutical industry trying to expand their markets, but it is also a product of the "popularization of symptoms and diagnoses" (Conrad, 2007, p. 67), spread through popular media, books, and lay organizations. Feedback dynamics between individuals seeking diagnoses and markets for empowering people through diagnoses and treatments thereof all constitute fundamental mechanisms of the diagnostic expansion. People's pursuit of a diagnosis fuels the engine of medicalization and in terms of adult ADHD, it might be the most influential factor. Thus, medicalization is rather a product of collective action than a consequence of "medical imperialism" (Conrad & Potter, 2000). This development points to a fundamental shift in how we as researchers need to examine the dynamics between diagnosis and the people being diagnosed, how to understand both the stigmatizing and legitimizing effect of diagnosis, and how to navigate in the paradox of both seeing diagnosis as an agent of social control and acknowledging that people increasingly demand diagnosis and welcome medical treatment.

Concluding remarks

The stories of ADHD presented in this chapter illustrate the complexity of understanding what ADHD is and how ADHD has emerged as a diagnostic category. ADHD is accepted as a psychiatric diagnosis and has been included in the diagnostic manuals for decades. Several scholars demonstrate how ADHD is caused by impairment in the executive functioning of the brain, and claim that behaviour connected to ADHD can be traced centuries back in time. Not everyone, however, subscribes to this story of ADHD and some researchers state that psychiatric diagnoses such as ADHD are not indicators of objective conditions but rather products of socio-political factors. It is argued that psychiatric diagnoses are socially and culturally situated, reflecting, and reinforcing contemporary ideas about the human in general and mental illness in particular.

The consequence of diagnosis, therefore, is also debated and while some view the diagnosis and the following treatment as a source of help for people suffering from a medical condition, others consider it a specious and damaging label, harming people who do not fit into our narrow conceptions of normality. The different explanations of ADHD are interpreted by many, ranging from Thom Hartmann (1994), who contends that hyperactive people genetically are hunters who have been left behind in modern society, to those like Conrad (2007), who believe that hyperactivity is a consequence of a high-performance and drug culture, continuously demanding more of people. Biopsychosocial approaches to ADHD try to mediate between the dichotomous viewpoints of ADHD as either a biologically or socially produced disorder, but are also critiqued for not situating ADHD in its historical contexts (Comstock, 2011; Davies, 2018). The approach is accused of failing to recognize how psychiatric knowledge is imbued with social values, and therefore still only offers one perspective of ADHD out of many. According to Smith (2012), what is alarming with all these different perspectives on ADHD is the unwillingness among scholars to accept the complexity of hyperactivity and the necessity of studying it from multiple perspectives. Pluralism and acceptance of various explanatory factors behind ADHD are much needed. As sociologist Nikolas Rose (2013) points out, few of us would dispute that neurological processes are involved in how we think feel, act, etc., but we also need to understand that mental illness is a matter of a living organism in its milieu (p. 33). Hinshaw and Scheffler (2014) also insist on acknowledging both biological, social, and cultural conceptions of ADHD and remind us that even if a disorder shows strong heritability, as ADHD does, social conditions still matter. Achievement pressures and demands of multitasking challenge everyone's ability to focus attention, but due to individual genetic difference, some people seem to be more affected than others. It is no coincidence that ADHD emerged in the context of mandatory schooling and that and rates of people diagnosed with ADHD have soared parallel to an increasing push for performance, since these developments have exhibited and elucidated the variation in people's attention span and inhibitory control.

To reduce ADHD to either a biological condition or a consequence of social and cultural changes is to leave out important research on ADHD. This chapter has attempted to outline some of the multiple investigations of ADHD – not to dig trenches or raise controversy, but rather to depict the different perspectives to the story of ADHD that each help illuminate what ADHD is and to illustrate how ADHD is undoubtedly a condition that raises much debate. Throughout the past decades – and even centuries – hyperactive and inattentive children have been the subject of medical, pedagogical, psychological, and sociological concern; each discipline insisting on different explanations for the type of behaviour. In this chapter, as indeed with this book, it is my ambition to embrace the pluralism of explanations of ADHD and to consider ADHD as a complex phenomenon that needs to be examined from multiple angles and with an understanding of its historical, political, and social context. Therefore, I recognize that all these different explanations exist and that they are all equally real. My interest is not to determine which explanation or story about ADHD holds more truth, but rather how people make use of these different explanations and what meanings they are inscribed with when used as ways of understanding oneself.

Acknowledgement

This chapter draws on work published in Nielsen, M. (2016). *Experiences of ADHD in adults: Morality, temporality and neurobiology*. Aalborg, Denmark: Aalborg Universitetsforlag. Reprinted by permission of Aalborg Universitetsforlag.

Notes

1 In Denmark, the new primary school reform from 2013 includes more physical activities in school, and the inactive teaching model might be changing.
2 Smith's example is taken from an American context; DTCA (direct-to consumer-advertisement) is not legal in Denmark.
3 Leo and Lacasse (2009) found the texts on the webpage in 2008. From my browsing through the webpage in spring 2019, I found no similar text.

References

American Psychiatric Association (APA). (2013). *Diagnostic and statistical manual of mental disorders: DSM-5*. Washington, DC: American Psychiatric Association.
Barkley, R. A. (2008). Commentary on excerpts of Crichton's chapter, on attention and its diseases. *Journal of Attention Disorders, 12*(3), 205–206.
Blaxter, M. (1978). Diagnosis as category and process: The case of alcoholism. *Social Science and Medicine, 12*, 9–17.
Bradley, C. (1950). Benzedrine® and Dexedrine® in the treatment of children's behavior disorders. *Pediatrics, 5*(24), 24–37.
Breggin, P. (1998). *Talking back to Ritalin*. Monroe, ME: Common Courage Press.
Comstock, E. J. (2011). The end of drugging children: Toward the genealogy of the ADHD subject. *Journal of the History of the Behavioral Sciences, 47*(1), 44–69.
Clarke, A. E., Shim, J. K., Mamo, L., Fosket, J. R., & Fishman, J. R. (2013). Biomedic alization: Technoscientific transformations of health, illness, and U.S. biomedicine. *American Sociological Review, 68*, 161–194.
Conrad, P. (1976). *Identifying hyperactive children: The medicalization of deviant behavior*. Lexington, MA: DC Heath & Company.
Conrad, P. (2007). *The medicalization of society: On the transformation of human conditions into treatable disorders*. Baltimore, MD: Johns Hopkins University Press.
Conrad, P., & Potter, D. (2000). From hyperactive children to ADHD adults: Observations on the expansion of medical categories. *Social Problems, 47*, 559–582.
Crichton, A. (1798/2008). An inquiry into the nature and origin of mental derange ment: On attention and its diseases. *Journal of Attention Disorders, 12*, 200–204.
Davies, A. (2018). Mapping the discourses of ADHD: The historical legacy. In M. Horton-Salway & A. Davies (Eds.), *The discourse of ADHD: Perspectives on attention deficit hyperactivity disorder* (pp. 27–68). Basingstoke, UK: Palgrave Macmillan.

DeGrandpre, R. (1999). *Ritalin nation: Rapid-fire culture and the transformation of human consciousness*. New York, NY: Norton.

Hartmann, T. (1994). *Attention deficit disorder: A different perception*. New York, NY: Underwood Books.

Hallowell, E. M., & Ratey, J. J. (1994). *Driven to distraction: Recognizing and coping with attention deficit disorder from childhood to adulthood*. New York, NY: Touchstone.

Hallowell, E. M., & Ratey, J. J. (2005). *Delivered from distraction: Getting the most out of life with attention deficit disorder*. New York, NY: Ballantine Books.

Hinshaw, S. P., & Scheffler, R. M. (2014). *The ADHD explosion: Myths, money, and today's push for performance*. New York, NY: Oxford University Press.

Kelly, K., & Ramundo, P. (1993). *You mean I'm not lazy, stupid, or crazy?! A self-help book for adults with attention deficit disorder*. New York, NY: Simon & Schuster.

Keohane, K., & Petersen, A. (2013). *The social pathologies of contemporary civilization*. Farnham, UK: Ashgate.

Kofod, E. H. (2017). From morality to pathology: A brief historization of contemporary Western grief practices and understandings. *Nordic Psychology*, *69*(1), 47–60.

Kutchins, H., & Kirk, S. (1997). *Making us crazy – DSM: The psychiatric bible and the creation of mental disorders*. Chicago, IL: University of Chicago Press.

Lange, W. K., Reichl, S., Lange, K. M., Tucha, L., & Tucha, O. (2010). The history of attention deficit hyperactivity disorder. *ADHD Attention Deficit Hyperactivity Disorder*, *2*(4), 241–255.

Leo, J., & Lacasse, J. (2009). The manipulation of data and attitudes about ADHD: A study of consumer advertisement. In S. Timimi & J. Leo (Eds.), *Rethinking ADHD: From brain to culture* (pp. 287–312). Basingstoke, UK: Palgrave Macmillan.

Mayes, R., & Rafalovich, A. (2007). Suffer the restless children: The evolution of ADHD and paediatric stimulant use, 1900–80. *History of Psychiatry*, *18*(4), 435–457.

Mercogliano, C. (2009). Canaries in the coal mine. In S. Timimi & J. Leo (Eds.), *Rethinking ADHD: From brain to culture* (pp. 382–397). Basingstoke, UK: Palgrave Macmillan.

Oxlund, B., &Whyte, S. R. (2014). Measuring and managing bodies in the later life course. *Population Ageing*, 7, 217–230.

Rafalovich, A. (2004). *Framing ADHD children: A critical examination of the history, discourse, and everyday experience of attention deficit/hyperactivity disorder*. Lanham, MD: Lexington Books.

Rose, N. (2013). What is diagnosis for? Talk given at the Institute of Psychiatry, King's College, London.

Rosenfeld, D., & Faircloth, C. A. (2006). Medicalized masculinities: The missing link? In D. Rosenfeld & C. A. Faircloth (Eds.) *Medicalized masculinities* (pp. 1–20). Philadelphia, PA: Temple University Press.

Smith, M. (2012). *Hyperactivity: The controversial history of ADHD*. London: Reaction Books.

Still, G. F. (1902/2006). Some abnormal physical conditions in children. *Journal of Attention Disorders*, *10*(2), 126–136.

Timimi, S. (2009). Why diagnosis of ADHD has increased so rapidly in the West: A cultural perspective. In S. Timimi & J. Leo (Eds.), *Rethinking ADHD: From brain to culture* (pp. 133–159). Basingstoke, UK: Palgrave Macmillan.

Timimi, S., & Leo, J. (2009). Introduction. In S. Timimi & J. Leo, (Eds.), *Rethinking ADHD: From brain to culture* (pp. 1–17). Basingstoke, UK: Palgrave Macmillan.

Wedge, M. (2015). *A disease called childhood: Why ADHD became an American epidemic*. New York, NY: Penguin.

Whitaker, R. (2010). *Anatomy of an epidemic: Magic bullets, psychiatric drugs, and the astonishing rise of mental illness in America*. New York, NY: Broadway Books.

Zola, I. K. (1972). Medicine as an institution of social control. *Sociological Review*, *20*, 487–504.

Chapter 3

What is a diagnosis?

> We have never been more aware of the arbitrary and constructed quality of psychiatric diagnoses, yet in an era characterized by the increasingly bureaucratic management of health care and an increasingly pervasive reductionism in the explanation of normal as well as pathological behavior, we have never been more dependent on them.
>
> (Rosenberg, 2006, p. 417)

In the previous chapter, I presented different explanations of ADHD and the emergence of the diagnosis. But what is a diagnosis? What role are diagnoses playing in contemporary health care? And how is a diagnosis "acting" and being acted upon? A diagnosis is the clinician's tool for classifying disorders and arranging treatment. As historian Charles E. Rosenberg writes in the epigraph to this chapter, diagnoses are fundamental for managing health care, despite the arbitrary quality of diagnoses. Similarly, Rose (2013) lists numerous ways diagnoses have come to function in our contemporary society: A diagnosis is a precondition for treatment and for financial coverage of its costs; a diagnosis gives access to social services; in clinical settings, a diagnosis is a central feature of patients' records; and for researchers, diagnoses make it possible to make estimates and predictions of incidence and prevalence. Besides the structuring function in institutional settings, researchers also describe how diagnoses become fundamental for people's interpretation of themselves and their suffering or difficulties. In this chapter, I present different perspectives on what a diagnosis is and how a biologization of the human being has changed our perception of being human in general and of mental illness in particular.

Diagnostic criteria and clinical guidelines

The diagnostic manuals' descriptions of and criteria for diagnoses are clearly central to our conceptions of what a diagnosis is and how impairment and human suffering is understood. In the case of ADHD, the disorder is listed in both the American Psychiatric Association's *Diagnostic and Statistical Manual of Mental Disorders* (DSM-5) and the World Health Organization's *International Classification of Diseases* (ICD-11) as a neurodevelopmental disorder. For each new edition of the two diagnostic systems, their descriptions of ADHD are becoming more alike and today are almost identical, as shown below.

The ICD-11, released in 2018 and expected to be implemented by its member states within the coming years, describes ADHD as follows:

> Attention deficit hyperactivity disorder is characterized by a persistent pattern (at least 6 months) of inattention and/or hyperactivity-impulsivity, with onset during the developmental period, typically early to mid-childhood. The degree of inattention and hyperactivity-impulsivity is outside the limits of normal variation expected for age and level of intellectual functioning and significantly interferes with academic, occupational, or social functioning. Inattention refers to significant difficulty in sustaining attention to tasks that do not provide a high level of stimulation or frequent rewards, distractibility and problems with organization. Hyperactivity refers to excessive motor activity and difficulties with remaining still, most evident in structured situations that require behavioural self-control. Impulsivity is a tendency to act in response to immediate stimuli, without deliberation or consideration of the risks and consequences. The relative balance and the specific manifestations of inattentive and hyperactive-impulsive characteristics varies across individuals, and may change over the course of development. In order for a diagnosis of disorder the behaviour pattern must be clearly observable in more than one setting.
>
> (WHO, 2018)

The DSM-5, released in 2013, describes ADHD as follows:

> *Inattention* manifests behaviorally in ADHD as wandering off task, lacking persistence, having difficulty sustaining focus, and being disorganized and is not due to defiance or lack of comprehension. *Hyperactivity* refers to excessive motor activity (such as a child running about) when it is not appropriate, or excessive fidgeting, tapping, or talkativeness. In adults, hyperactivity may manifest as extreme restlessness or wearing others out with their activity. *Impulsivity* refers to hasty actions that occur in the moment without forethought and that have high potential for harm to the individual (e.g., darting into the street without looking).
>
> (APA, 2013, p. 61)

Criteria for getting the ADHD diagnosis, according to DSM-5, is a positive response to the following list of elaborate symptom descriptions:

Inattention:

a. Often fails to give close attention to details or makes careless mistakes in schoolwork, at work, or during other activities (e.g. overlooks or misses details, work is inaccurate).
b. Often has difficulty sustaining attention in tasks or play activities (e.g. has difficulty remaining focused during lectures, conversations, or lengthy reading).
c. Often does not seem to listen when spoken to directly (e.g. mind seems elsewhere, even in the absence of any obvious distraction).
d. Often does not follow through on instructions and fails to finish school-work, chores, or duties in the workplace (e.g. starts tasks but quickly loses focus and is easily sidetracked).
e. Often has difficulty organizing tasks and activities (e.g. difficulty managing sequential tasks; difficulty keeping materials and belongings in order; messy, disorganized work; has poor time management; fails to meet deadlines).
f. Often avoids, dislikes, or is reluctant to engage in tasks that require sustained mental effort (e.g. schoolwork or homework; for older adolescents and adults, preparing reports, completing forms, reviewing lengthy papers).
g. Often loses things necessary for tasks or activities (e.g. school materials, pencils, books, tools, wallets, keys, paperwork, eyeglasses, mobile telephones).
h. Is often easily distracted by extraneous stimuli (for older adolescents and adults, may include unrelated thoughts).
i. Is often forgetful in daily activities (e.g. doing chores, running errands; for older adolescents and adults, returning calls, paying bills, keeping appointments).

Hyperactivity and impulsivity:

a. Often fidgets with or taps hands or feet or squirms in seat.
b. Often leaves seat in situations when remaining seated is expected (e.g. leaves his or her place in the classroom, in the office or other workplace, or in other situations that require remaining in place).
c. Often runs about or climbs in situations where it is inappropriate. (Note: In adolescents or adults, may be limited to feeling restless.).
d. Often unable to play or engage in leisure activities quietly.
e. Is often "on the go", acting as if "driven by a motor" (e.g. is unable to be or uncomfortable being still for an extended time, such as in restaurants, meetings; may be experienced by others as being restless or difficult to keep up with).

f.   Often talks excessively.
g.   Often blurts out an answer before a question has been completed (e.g. completes people's sentences; cannot wait for their turn in conversation).
h.   Often has difficulty waiting his or her turn (e.g. while waiting in line).
i.   Often interrupts or intrudes on others (e.g. butts into conversations, games, or activities; may start using other people's things without asking or receiving permission; for adolescents and adults, may intrude into or take over what others are doing).

At least six (five for adolescents and adults) of the listed symptoms for inattention and hyperactivity-impulsivity respectively need to be present to a degree that is "inconsistent with developmental level and that negatively impacts directly on social and academic/occupational activities" (APA, 2013, p. 59f). Moreover, the symptoms need to have persisted for at least six months in order to avoid temporary problems of life crises to interfere with the manifestation of symptoms. Another related criterion is the presence of the symptoms causing the impairment before the age of 12. Furthermore, the specific behavioural difficulties need to be present in multiple settings and there must be clinical evidence of significant impairment and performance issues in social, educational, or work contexts. As the listed diagnostic descriptions show, the symptoms need to manifest themselves often and they need to be assessed as causing severe difficulties. But when is "often" often enough, as it is stated in each listed symptom description? And when are the symptoms sufficiently affecting social and academic activities for a diagnosis to be given? Demarcating on a continuum what is "normal" behaviour and behaviour related to ADHD is ultimately based on convention and psychiatric evaluation and therefore also based on local conceptions of normality (Hinshaw & Scheffler, 2014).

According to the clinical guidelines for diagnosing adults offered by the Danish Health Authority, diagnosis is given based on a questionnaire completed by the patient and a thorough interview with patient and relatives, both addressing problems experienced during childhood and adulthood. Anamnesis should contain systematically collected information about the individual's development and psychiatric symptoms and accompanying difficulties from early childhood until adulthood and possibly substance abuse. Moreover, information about the individual's health, social, and economic status and educational and occupational background should be collected (Sundhedsstyrelsen, 2015). In order to collect the preferred information, the adult ADHD self-report scale (ASRS), a questionnaire that in a structured way collects self-reported information about the patient's symptoms, is recommended for initial assessment. Diva 2.0, a semi-structured interview guide that aims to systematically collect information about the patient's symptoms, is also recommended. In terms of treatment, The Danish Health Authority recommends methylphenidate or lisdexamfetamine, both central nervous system stimulants. If the patient is considered to benefit from it, medical treatment is combined with cognitive behavioural therapy. Psych education, where the patient is taught about the diagnosis, is listed as good practice. According to the guidelines, evidence shows an effect on ADHD symptoms and functional capacity from pharmaceutical treatment and despite reports of unwanted side effects, the advantages of the treatment are considered to exceed the disadvantages.

While studies of ADHD estimate a 2.5–5.3 per cent prevalence in the adult population (APA, 2013, p. 61; Barkley, Murphy, & Fischer, 2008, p. 17), there are considerable differences in numbers of people diagnosed with ADHD across countries, which might be accounted for by both different diagnostic practices and by cultural variations in attitudes towards or interpretations of behaviour. For example, numbers of people diagnosed with ADHD in countries using the ICD have traditionally been lower than in countries following the DSM (Hinshaw & Scheffler, 2014, p. 123). Patterns also show that rates of diagnoses are higher in countries with a certain level of economic development, perhaps revealing different priorities in terms of how to enhance conditions for the population (Hinshaw & Scheffler, 2014, p. 135).[1] Within countries, rates of people diagnosed may also vary, and research in the United States demonstrates that rates of ADHD diagnoses in different ethnic populations differ among, for example, Latino and Caucasian populations (APA, 2013, p. 62). In Denmark, research on geographical differences across regions shows large variations of ADHD in the municipalities despite tax-financed and free access to health care. Differences in sociodemographic composition explain little of regional variation and results rather indicate that accessibility to diagnostic resources accounts for the variation in ADHD incidence (Madsen, Ersbøll, Olsen, Parner, & Obel, 2015; Wallach-Kildemoes, Skovgaard, Thielen, Pottegård, & Mortensen, 2015). It seems, therefore, that perceptions of who is diagnosed with ADHD, access to diagnostic resources, as well as regional diagnostic practices are all decisive factors in explaining some of the variation in numbers of diagnoses of ADHD within countries.

What is diagnosis for?

To ask what a diagnosis is for might seem odd, but depending on the perspective, the answer may vary. Most obviously, diagnoses define and describe what is considered beyond the "normal". Throughout the history of psychiatry as a discipline, doctors have defined the boundaries between the "normal" and "abnormal" and determined which measures should be taken in terms of treatment. Every psychiatric diagnosis, notwithstanding the means used for assessing and explaining the behaviours, emotions, or sensations, is determined based on a social evaluation and therefore always subject to contestation. In the case of ADHD, one could ask what levels of attention are appropriate, why this particular skill should be evaluated within the psychiatric domain, and where to draw the line between notions of the pathological and ideas about enhancement? When does psychiatry treat genuine distress and when is psychiatry contributing to the creation of a culture focusing too much on academic performance and leaving too little room for difference? Such questions remain central when discussing what diagnoses are for. Deviance will always be context dependent, and psychiatric diagnoses will reflect different institutional practices and cultural conceptions of normality. As numerous researchers have described, diagnoses tend to emerge and disappear again, depended on sociopolitical, moral, and cultural streams, and will therefore always be a product of negotiated processes. Only 30 years ago, homosexuality was considered pathological, and looking even further back in time, masturbation was on the same list (Conrad, 2007; Rosenberg, 2006). To examine these cases today illustrate the normative aspects of diagnoses, and as patterns of cultural norms and clinical guidelines change, so will different aspects of human behaviour and emotions be considered pathological and evaluated within a diagnostic framework.

Establishing what she calls a sociology of diagnoses, Annemarie Jutel (2011) argues that diagnoses are social constructions that provide "a cultural expression of what a given society is prepared to accept as normal and what it feels should be treated" (p. 3). Overall, three circumstances determine if a condition is classified as a disease and listed as a diagnosis: First, it must be recognized as undesirable; second, technology needs to be able to discern it; and lastly, a collective will to assimilate the condition into the spectrum of diseases needs to be present. That diagnoses are constructed, however, does not mean that they are not real, but rather that their existence is bound to what is defined as problematic. In that perspective, Jutel (2011) emphasizes, diagnoses are concepts formed by biology, technology, the social, the political, and the lived. Diagnoses capture a reality despite their fluid nature of that reality, and to exemplify her point, Jutel refers to an illustrative description by Mirowsky and Ross (1989), who describe diagnoses as "star constellations in the sky". These formations are truly present, but the meaning of them is shaped by how we assemble them in recognizable patterns. Like constellations of stars, symptoms are linked together to create a diagnostic pattern, and "a collective cultural position determines which symptoms we will see, which we will brush off as insignificant, how we make sense of what is there, and what social consequences the diagnosis will convey" (Jutel, 2011, p. 61).

Besides differentiating between the "normal" and "abnormal", identifying the problem, and directing treatment, diagnoses also function as a structuring tool, organizing not only behaviours and emotions but also professions and institutions. Mol (2002) and Brinkmann (2014) point to the multiple players enacting and "doing" diagnoses, ranging from words, buildings, systems, institutions, etc. From this perspective, diagnoses function as boundary objects (Bowker & Star, 2000) that enable very different disciplines and actors to communicate about the same object – even if each actor defines the object of study differently. Whether it is the patient, doctor, social worker, insurance company, or policymaker interpreting what ADHD entails, the term itself renders conversation possible. From one institution to another, the diagnosis as a boundary object travels in administrative structures and is referred to in political and juridical evaluations. Diagnoses, thus, have a fundamental role in organizing psychiatric knowledge and allocating research funding, just as academic journals are often organized into specific diagnostic interests (Rose, 2013). There are, for example, academic journals only dealing with research on ADHD, and factors such as comorbidity or patterns of symptoms that do not fit into the existing diagnostic categories may challenge the order of professional communication and research. As such, diagnoses are part of a complex network of actors, institutions, and technologies that each make use of diagnoses for very different purposes. In Denmark, for example, a newly implemented primary school reform, which promotes inclusion of children with special needs into the mainstream school system, have raised a debate over whether or not children with diagnoses such as ADHD should automatically be accompanied with economic resources for pedagogical backup. The diagnosis therefore has a practical value in terms of administrative decisions concerning potential measures and policymaking (Arnfred & Langager, 2015).

Another, yet related, central feature when discussing what diagnoses are and what they are for is the aspect of specificity. Historian Charles Rosenberg (2002) describes the change in psychiatry when focus shifted from etiology to symptoms and the discipline started to understand various forms of human suffering in terms of specific diagnostic categories. From his analysis of technological breakthroughs in medical history, Rosenberg outlines the dilemma in what he calls "disease specificity" and the idea that idiosyncratic human beings can fit into constructed and constricting ideal-typical diagnostic categories. This disease specificity is based on the notion that diseases are entities existing outside their manifestation in particular individuals, and the context in which the symptoms appear is neglected

(p. 237). As not only medicine but also society has become more and more specialized and bureaucratic, there is an increased need for specific diagnoses with inherent treatment plans that can easily administer each course of disease. As Rosenberg notes, human beings have always used words to signify what was considered pathological, and throughout history doctors have had a special role when distinguishing between different diseases and in mastering the medical vocabulary. But whereas diseases were previously considered to be fluid and transient, and could follow very different trajectories, our perception of diseases are much more specific and categorical today. Part of this transformation in how to think of diseases is promoted by technical developments as for example thermometers, X-ray technologies, microscopes, and electrocardiograms (EKGs) that in different ways made it possible to measure diseases in units and represent them visually (p. 243). Being able to identify diseases concretely and observing them as something tangible, changed the fluid and nonspecific ideas about diseases by the beginning of the twentieth century, and today the idea of disease specificity dominates both the somatic and psychiatric fields. Despite being contested by several scholars, who question the epistemological as well as the ontological status of diagnoses, these categories have become central in defining the agreed-upon knowledge about diseases as specific entities. We think of diagnoses as separate entities and they function as such when they travel outside the clinic in terms of both rights and privileges and in terms of identity making and notions of responsibility.

Creating mental illness

The debate over the ontological status and comprehension of psychiatric diagnoses has many participants. One of them, and a particular critical voice, is sociologist Alan Horwitz. In his book *Creating Mental Illness* (2002), Horwitz criticizes the so-called diagnostic psychiatry for not differentiating between genuine mental diseases and cultural expressions of distress. From his 25-year study of mental disorders, he identifies a change in both mental health professionals' and patients' understanding of mental illness and directs his critique towards the publication of the DSM-III, which marked a revolution in the professional conception of mental illness. What happened with the DSM-III was a change from a holistic, etiological approach to diagnosing people, often based on psychoanalytic theory, to a symptom-based approach, in which certain clusters of symptoms are considered to indicate distinct underlying diseases. Although the diagnostic psychiatry officially acknowledges that no biomarker can identify mental disorders and that psychiatry is therefore bound to diagnose patients on the basis of clinical observations, Horwitz (2002) claims that the underlying assumption in the diagnostic system still emphasizes organic pathologies rather than accepting that there are often a variety of factors behind mental disorders. The primary problem with diagnostic psychiatry, therefore, is how biological explanatory models dominate our conception of distress, and "locate the pathological qualities of psychological conditions in the physical properties of brains, not in the symbolic systems of minds" (p. 3). According to Horwitz, we need to differentiate between genuine mental diseases, which are "conditions where symptoms indicate underlying internal dysfunctions" (p. 15), and mental illnesses, which refer to "whatever a particular social group defines as such" (p. 15). To address the two similarly is simply mistaken. Horwitz argues that mental diseases such as schizophrenia, bipolar disorders, and other psychoses fit the premise of a diagnostic psychiatry, since they show dysfunctions in mechanisms regulating perception and thinking. Mental illnesses, on the contrary, do not fit into the schema because of their cultural dependency. According to Horwitz, that does not mean that people with mental illnesses are not suffering, but rather that they need to be understood as ontologically different to mental diseases.

Like Rosenberg, who describes the historical emergence of disease specificity, Horwitz lists several factors behind the success of the diagnostic psychiatry and the influential idea of specific disease entities. For one thing, research-oriented psychiatrists needed specific cases to study and therefore embraced a system that allowed them to more clearly demarcate different mental disorders, to compare cases, and to generalize beyond research sites (Mayes & Horwitz, 2005, p. 256). In the clinical room, psychiatrists needed specific categories to obtain reimbursements for their services (Horwitz, 2002, p. 74). Politically, it suited the administrative climate to focus more on specific illnesses with specific treatment options rather than on broad complex social problems (p. 77), and insurance companies increasingly demanded diagnoses and treatment that were demonstratively effective and financially accountable (Mayes & Horwitz, 2005, p. 254). Similarly, lay advocacy groups, fighting for the rights of people with mental illnesses, welcomed the idea that mental illnesses are brain-based disorders caused by biological factors, since it rejected the theory that mental illness is caused by poor parenting and traumatic experiences (Horwitz, 2002, p. 77). And last but not least, psychiatry was facing a major dilemma, as psychotherapy was not only growing in popularity, but was also increasingly performed by psychologists who undercut psychiatrists in terms of price. Psychiatry therefore had to decide how to demonstrate the legitimacy of their profession if they were leaving psychotherapy to other professions. Here, it is argued, the diagnostic psychiatry with its focus on neurobiology and drug treatment was the solution to strengthening psychiatry as a profession (Mayes & Horwitz, 2005, p. 257). Overall, with the DSM-III, psychiatry shifted from a dynamic understanding of mental illnesses to a biological understanding that stresses brain chemistry and drug treatment and supersedes the psychosocial understanding of mental illness that had dominated for decades.

Horwitz, 2002) represents the critical statement, shared by many scholars, that people who become depressed or anxious "react in *appropriate* ways to their environments" (p. 14, italics in original), and that they would not be mentally disordered if their disturbing social circumstances changed. According to Horwitz, the introduction of diagnostic psychiatry has ultimately led to an overestimation of the prevalence of mental disorders and improper treatment of people experiencing mental distress. Like Conrad (2007), who describes a medicalization of human phenomena, Horwitz (2002) points to the continuous inclusion of new types of distress into the diagnostic manuals and critiques the increasing comprehension of all kinds of suffering as caused by biological dysfunctions in the brain. As part of this argument, Horwitz highlights a central concern, namely that even if people's reactions to stress vary only slightly across time and place, the meaning people ascribe to these reactions, notions of what causes the reactions, and the help people seek to ease the suffering has changed dramatically within the last couple of decades. The proliferation of mental disorders illustrates how a medicalized disease framework increasingly encompasses more and more problematic psychological conditions. Too many of the conditions represented in the DSM reflect expectable reactions to stressful conditions and general human unhappiness and dissatisfaction. Judged from the numbers of included diagnoses in the DSM from the first edition, which was a rather slim volume, to the latest much heavier edition, Horwitz may have a point. One might ask whether we are witnessing an epidemic of distress and genuine mental diseases, if we tend to pathologize increasingly more aspects of human life, or if we are becoming better at identifying suffering that was previously left unnoticed. Nevertheless, it is evident that the diagnostic manuals contain more and more diagnoses and cover more and more of the human existence than ever before.

In the case of ADHD, as I outlined in the previous chapter, the diagnosis is accused by critics for being a consequence of the medicalization of behaviour and underperformance rather than a genuine mental disease. Following Horwitz (2002), ADHD might reflect an expectable reaction to the changing conditions in modern life, and people experiencing symptoms related to ADHD might react in appropriate ways to the challenges they meet. If expectations in school, at work, and changes in level of activity favour certain kinds of behaviour, ADHD-related behaviour intensifies. And if we at the same time witness a diminishing of tolerance for and appreciation of the diversity of human life, this kind of behaviour becomes inappropriate and will eventually be subjected to medicalization. Together, these analyses reveal some of the processes of social control and institutional bureaucratization as drivers for pathologization and medicalization of behaviour. However, the analyses primarily point to the different engines of disease specificity and the development of medical categories, and less to the processes of how individuals internalize, interpret, and live with these medical and therapeutic descriptions of their behaviour, emotions, and sensations, and how, or rather whether, they become an integrated part of their subjectivity. These aspects, as I will show in the following section, also work as drivers of medicalization.

Putting a name to it

Rose (2013) claims that diagnosing is performative. It is a process in which the doctor solves his own problem (he must react satisfactorily to the patient's request and leave the patient with a feeling of being treated in an acceptable manner) and solves the patient's problem (experiences of suffering) by directing treatment. Diagnoses function as a way of systemizing experiences in institutional settings but diagnoses also affect the individual whose experiences are systemized. They transform an "unorganized illness", unconnected symptoms, and experiences of suffering into an understandable "organized illness" (Conrad, 2007, p. 46). Or as Rosenberg (2002) notes, pointing to the standardization process that transforms experiences into categories within institutions, "it helps makes experience machine readable" (p. 257). These categories and interpretations of human distress may offer new insights and valuable narratives, but they might also stigmatize or reduce the complexity of human experience to a simple description. What used to be diffuse bodily sensations or emotional difficulties are analysed, categorized, and labelled within a diagnostic framework that offers a specific narrative to the suffering. Rose (2013) similarly describes how a diagnosis enables the doctor to organize the patient's history into a treatable condition and how the diagnosis reframes troubles into an illness, thus providing a framework for understanding the past and for orienting to the future for the patient. Likewise, the patient's abstract experiences and difficulties are reinterpreted from being understood as perhaps personal inadequacies into a treatable condition. The built-in narrative in the diagnosis renders possible a much more concrete way of understanding and talking about suffering, and even if a diagnosis sometimes predicts a life with chronic illness, it is welcomed by many because of its ability to transform experiences into a comprehensible entity.

While a diagnosis provides structure and distinguishes the pathological from the normal, a diagnosis also potentially rearranges identity. For example, Martin (2007) argues that a diagnosis brings about new subject positions. Once diagnosed, the individual is no longer a person with life problems but a person living under the description of the particular diagnosis. As a transformative moment, when the individual embarks on, in Goffman's (1959) words, a "moral career" as someone with a diagnosis, the diagnosis potentially changes self-perceptions as well as others' perceptions of the diagnosed (Novas & Rose, 2000). Therefore, diagnoses are not just products of culture, they are also producers of it. In Rosenberg's (2002) words, diagnoses have become "indisputable social actors, real inasmuch as we have believed in them and acted individually and collectively on those beliefs" (p. 240). They "act" on people and despite their constructed quality, they have real, social implications. From her own experience of going through a diagnostic process, Jutel (2011) describes how the diagnosis came to play an important role in the way she understands her life and illness. The diagnosis conferred a new identity, as she, in the moment of the diagnosis, "became someone with an autoimmune disorder" (p. xii). To be that someone may remove the individual from the isolation of his or her suffering and provide the person with a new collective identity together with others suffering from the same condition. Referencing Talcott Parsons' notion of the sick role, Jutel (2011) argues that "being diagnosed gives permission to be ill", and once diagnosed, the suffering person is no longer blamed for failing social expectations, but is instead treated for a disease.

A diagnosis, thus, can both stigmatize and legitimize conditions dependent on how the diagnosis is commonly perceived. As an example, people diagnosed with fibromyalgia often ambiguously welcome the diagnosis, since a psychiatric diagnosis is taken as a denial of the patient's experience of physical pain. On the one hand, receiving the diagnosis gives relief because it validates the suffering and gives a sense of credibility, but on the other hand, the psychiatric diagnosis does not necessarily cover what the patients believe to be a physical disease (Jutel, 2011, p. 78). Hence, the legitimacy of the diagnosis relies on whether it corresponds with what society and the patient recognize as a legitimate disease or a valid explanation, and whether the patient accepts the narrative offered by the diagnosis. Similarly, the degree to which the diagnosis is incorporated into and rearranges identity depends on whether the diagnosis is accepted by the patient. Diagnoses carry different moral values and especially psychiatric diagnoses may generate stigma, such as social exclusion, prejudices concerning the person's ability to think and act rationally, etc. For that reason, diagnoses are sometimes rejected by the diagnosed, who do not wish to be associated with a particular diagnosis.

As I will show in Chapter 4, adults diagnosed with ADHD often welcome the diagnosis as a legitimization of their problems and an official explanation of their difficulties. In research, we might point to the arbitrary construction of the diagnosis and emphasize diagnosis as a pragmatic tool for treating suffering, but from the patient's perspective, diagnosis become much more than that. An ADHD diagnosis brings about new ways of understanding oneself and of managing everyday practices, and it might even become used as a kind of identity marker. Diagnosis structures experiences by offering a specific narrative to the suffering and in Chapter 4, I analyse how this structuring effect unfolds in my interlocutors' lives and engagement with the diagnosis. The fact that diagnosis potentially offers identities, legitimacy, and access to resources, explains the gravity in the battle over diagnoses. As also noted by Conrad (2007) and Horwitz (2002), Jutel (2011) points to lay social movements' advocacy for specific diagnoses in search of explanation and legitimization as an illustration of how diagnoses have become the centre of battles not only inside psychiatry but also in society. The submissive patient has become a minority among those pursuing a diagnosis (p. 69), and diagnoses have increasingly become the subject of negation and disputes of recognition.

Living in a diagnostic culture

As demonstrated in Chapter 2, societal changes have brought about transformations in the cultural idioms for communication of discontent, and traditional ways of expressing suffering are being replaced by a psychiatric understanding of human distress (Scheper-Hughes & Lock, 1987). Pointing to the rising numbers of diagnoses in the psychiatric manuals, the institutional use of diagnoses beyond the psychiatric system, the growing number of people receiving psychiatric diagnoses, and people's own use of diagnostic categories when understanding their suffering, researchers suggest that we are living in a diagnostic culture (Brinkmann, Peterson, Kofod, & Birk, 2014). A diagnostic culture is characterized by the circulation of psychiatric diagnoses and categories that not only professionals (doctors, psychologists, psychiatrists, etc.), but also laypeople and the public use in order to understand life problems and human deviance within many different social practices. TV series often portray characters with different psychiatric diagnoses and people generally know about central patterns of symptom for several psychiatric diagnoses. The popular media have put diagnoses on the agenda, and diagnostic tests have become a frequent feature in various kinds of magazines. The cover of a Danish newspaper, for example, asked: "Do you have a psychiatric disorder without knowing it? Symptoms you might overlook", thereby encouraging people to evaluate themselves following a diagnostic logic. From my own teaching at the University of Copenhagen, I sometimes ask my students if they have ever taken an online diagnostic test and normally about half of the students raise their hand. In a time when still more and more aspects of the human existence are interpreted through a diagnostic logic, diagnoses seem to invade our everyday life. The diagnostic language infiltrates everyday language when we talk about being depressed, when we are sad or disappointed, being schizophrenic when we are having mixed feelings about something, and being manic when we are eagerly occupied with a task.

In his book *Diagnostic Cultures*, Brinkmann (2016) critiques the pervasiveness of the diagnostic gaze and calls for a more diverse and inclusive approach to understanding human suffering. While the diagnostic language spreads, other ways of understanding the human being become less influential and the overall palette of understanding narrows. As a consequence, our tools for addressing human suffering are limited correspondingly. Across cultures and through any historical era, human discontent is shaped, given expression, and responded to using certain languages and explanations (Rose, 2006). Experts have always had the authority to define and intervene when people have sought professional assistance in fragile periods of their lives, but when options for seeking advice, help, and comfort is limited to a certain kind of profession or explanation, our vocabulary for expressing and ability to understand existential problems in a nuanced way is threatened. According to Brinkmann (2016), we risk losing vital resources of self-understanding if we only know how to manage and relieve people from their suffering by pathologizing it. When existential, political, and moral concerns are interpreted within a diagnostic framework, their historical and social origin is lost, and we miss not only the contextual factors behind the individual's experiences of distress but also the means for addressing the problem.

In a similar vein, Kleinman and Kleinman (1991) point to the risk of delegitimizing expressions of, for example, moral commentary or political performance by transforming misery resulting from political calamity into psychiatric diagnoses. Examples of people who never wanted to align their experiences with medical descriptions, but whose experiences have been pathologized, bear witness to the power of diagnoses on both an individual level and as a structuring and governing tool in society. Another contemporary and controversial example is the debate over whether or not complicated and prolonged grief should be a diagnosis. Historically, grief has been practised, interpreted, and experienced within a framework of religion and morality, but since the beginning of the twentieth century, we have gradually come to understand experiences of grief from a psychological and psychiatric perspective (Kofod, 2017). In relation to the release of the new diagnostic manuals, scholars have discussed potentials and perils connected to grief being a diagnosis, and while some favour a diagnosis in order to direct precise therapy, others are worried about the increasing medicalization of emotions. However, in the most recent edition, the ICD-11 included "prolonged grief disorder", while the DSM-5 suggests the diagnosis "persistent complex bereavement disorder" should be further studied (Kofod, 2017). From moralization to pathologization – each perspective involves limited conceptual frameworks for understanding, and each explanatory model we use for understanding suffering leads to certain interventions. As Brinkmann (2016) writes, the perspective from which you look, determines what you see. If you have a hammer, everything looks like a nail. If you have a diagnostic manual, everything will look like a symptom (p. 129). What the critical position in describing and mapping the diagnostic culture offers is suspicion of simplistic and isolated ideas of diagnoses explaining people's problems and encourages us to expand our conceptions of human suffering.

A neurochemical era

The diagnostic gaze is accused of reducing human experiences to an inhuman disease, but the explanatory models used for understanding sufferings are also critiqued. While the theory of a chemical imbalance in the brain as the cause of mental illness has been subject to critique and is now widely rejected, a general biologization of mental illness still strongly prevails.

Neuroscientists are now examining subjects that traditionally have been studied from psychological, anthropological, philosophical, and religious angles and the humanities are increasingly inspired by neuroscientific knowledge about how human nature is shaped by the structure and functions of the brain (Rose & Abi-Rached, 2013). Similarly, research on ADHD reflects a tremendous interest in the neurobiological mechanisms of the disorder and as outlined in Chapter 2, medicalization is transferring a variety of human phenomena into the medical domain. More recently, the concept of biomedicalization has been introduced by scholars to demonstrate the epistemic shift from a clinical to a molecular gaze (Clarke, Mamo, Fosket, Fishman, & Shim, 2010). New technoscientific changes in the practices of contemporary biomedicine constitute this shift, as new technologies intervene not only in the organization of medical care but also in how we think about the human being and life itself (p. 2). Biomedicalization, just as medicalization, is concerned with eliminating pathology but it is also concerned with managing, engineering, reshaping, and enhancing the human being based on new biomedical innovations (p. 11). A critical question, therefore, concerns to what degree individuals have access to and are tempted by the possibilities offered by new scientific discoveries (Singh & Rose, 2006, p. 97). Are, for example, individuals who experience an overwhelming pressure of expectation, who are in a vulnerable situation in life, or a disadvantaged position in society more limited from or more inclined to search for help through the possibilities of medical developments?

The question of how biomedicalization processes and neurobiological knowledge changes the way we think about the human being in general and (mental) illnesses specifically is extensively discussed within a wide range of research disciplines. The current debate provokes questions about how we as laypersons engage with this type of knowledge and if it has produced a shift in everyday conceptions of the self. The implications concern, then, both how people engage with these new possibilities at the individual level (as bodies, selves, and consumers), and collectively (as health social movements and patient groups) (Clarke et al., 2010, p. 11). In an article reviewing empirical investigations of how neuroscientific knowledge affects lay understandings of personhood, psychologists Cliodhna O'Connor and Helene Joffe (2013) conclude that neuroscientific ideas become integrated in our understandings of selfhood and that especially people who have been through a diagnostic process adapt the neuroscientific knowledge. According to the review, some of the most radical research results suggest that neuroscientific insights "will fundamentally alter the dynamic between personal identity, responsibility and free will" (Illes & Racine, 2005, p. 14), and that "neuroimaging has contributed to a fundamental change in how we think of ourselves and our fellow persons" (Farah, 2012, p. 575). It is further suggested that neuroscientific knowledge is "propelling humanity toward a radical reshaping of our lives, families, societies, cultures, governments, economies, art, leisure, religion – absolutely everything that's pivotal to humankind's existence" (Lynch, 2009, p. 7). O'Connor and Joffe (2013), however, also conclude that the effect of neuroscientific knowledge on people's conception of selfhood is sometimes overestimated and that neuroscientific knowledge is assimilated into our existing social and psychological ideas about selfhood in ways that "perpetuate rather than challenge existing modes of understanding" (p. 262).

Studies examining the impact of neurobiological explanations of ADHD in public and private discourses come to similar conclusions (Bröer & Heerings, 2013; Danforth & Navarro, 2001; Horton-Salway, 2011). Sociologists Christian Bröer and Marjolijn Heerings (2013) found that a neurobiological discourse dominates public discourses about ADHD in Holland, while personal discourses encompass more various descriptions of ADHD ranging from sociological to spiritual portrayals of the disorder. Researcher in discursive psychology, Mary Horton-Salway (2011), found two overall repertoires representing stories about ADHD in the UK newspapers: first, a biological repertoire that describes ADHD as a brain disorder and justifies medical treatment for ADHD; and second, a psychosocial repertoire that support moral judgments about the so-called "sick society" and criticizes medicalization processes for the diagnostic labelling of bad behaviour. Generally, it seems that, similar to the two main explanations of the emergence of ADHD as described in Chapter 2, research in public discourses identifies both a position explaining ADHD as a neurobiological disorder and a position explaining ADHD as a product of social and cultural factors.

A shift in thinking about the human being

Rose and Abi-Rached (2013) outline how the social sciences have shifted back and forth between a biologization and a psychologization of the human being. In the eighteenth-century's racial sciences, a biologization of the human being dominated scientific understandings of human nature, but the period was followed by an intense psychologization of the human throughout the first half of the twentieth century. And now, paradoxically, we witness a return to the biological explanation of human nature in the form of the influence of neuroscience. Horwitz (2002) makes a similar analysis, stating that the emphasis on the biological explanations of mental disorders is a reappearance of earlier biological thinking in psychiatry (p. 132). Especially after the Second World War, biological theories became associated with eugenic programmes and a reactionary political climate, and the biological theories were therefore discredited. As a result, a period of what Horwtiz (2002) calls dynamic psychiatry came to dominate psychiatric thinking. Moreover, the anti-psychiatry ideology in the 1970s, represented in popular culture with movies like *One Flew Over the Cuckoo's Nest* (1975), criticized biological psychiatry for "creating the forms of damages and disordered selfhood that it claimed to explain" (Rose & Abi-Rached, 2013, p. 113). Today, the scientific landscape has shifted again, and the study of the brain and genetics again dominates psychiatry (Horwitz, 2002, p. 133). The accusations against psychiatry, however, have not gone silent and researchers such as Whitaker (2010) and psychiatrist David Healy (2012) criticize the pharmaceutical industry for doing more damage than good and for incorrectly explaining mental illness as the consequence of a chemical imbalance in the brain. Generally, however, a "regime of futurity" (Rose & Abi-Rached, 2013, p. 14), in which science wishes to govern the future, prevent illnesses, and tackle the burdens of mental disorders, has come to form our way of thinking.

So, what does this neurobiologization of the human entail? Rose and Abi-Rached (2013) claim that non-conscious neural processes are considered as constituents of moral action and that especially researchers and professionals working with mental health consider the brain as a target of self-improvement (p. 219). As they put it:

> We extend our hopes and fears over our biological bodies to that special organ of the brain; act upon the brain as on the body, to reform, cure, or improve ourselves; and have a new register to understand, speak and act upon ourselves – and on others – as the kinds of beings whose characteristics are shaped by neurobiology.
>
> (p. 223)

The concept of the brain's plasticity, however, is central. We acknowledge that human brains are both shaped by and shape their sociality and the neurobiological understanding of selfhood has not eliminated or rejected psychological understandings of selfhood, but the two approaches exist concurrently. With this in mind, we are expected to take moral responsibility for nurturing and optimizing the brain in the best way possible (p. 223). The brain in effect becomes the subject for interventions of various kinds.

The self in medical terms

Rose's (2003) analysis of "the neurochemical self" and how modern individuals have come to understand themselves in terms of their brains and bodies is highly referenced in sociological research on contemporary biomedicine. Inspired by Foucault's notions of governmentality, Rose (2003) claims that active and responsible citizens are obliged to constantly monitor their health and improve themselves in response to society's requirements and that pharmaceuticals have come to be the tool in these self-disciplining practices (p. 59). Pharmaceuticals "are entangled with certain conceptions of what human are or should be" (p. 59) and taking drugs becomes a practice of adapting behaviour in line with cultural norms.

While Rose (2003) introduces the "neurochemical self", anthropologist Janis Jenkins (2010) presents what she calls the "pharmaceutical self". Since the primary source of psychiatric treatment is psychopharmacology and because aggressive marketing of pharmaceuticals shapes the perception of subjects in need of treatment, Jenkins claims that we have become pharmaceutical selves. Based on her research on the treatment of psychoses, Jenkins examines the dialectic between what she calls the "pharmaceutical imaginary", which is the dimension of culture oriented towards pharmaceuticals as potentials for human life, and the "pharmaceutical self", which is the aspect of the self oriented toward pharmaceutical drugs (p. 23). According to Jenkins, individuals adopt the pharmaceutical imaginary of mental illnesses as caused by chemical imbalances and interpret themselves and their problems in light of this imaginary. According to Jenkins, subjectivity is not only a feature of individual experience, and it cannot be distinguished from its surroundings, but the self must be understood as the sum of processes by which the subject is oriented in the world and toward other people. As patients incorporate and take the idea of schizophrenia as a consequence of a chemical imbalance, schizophrenia as a form of subjectivity can only be understood as strongly intertwined with the idea of restoring the balance with psychopharmacology. Thus, both Rose and Jenkins address the consequences of neurobiological explanations not only for decisions about treatment but also how we think about ourselves. Similarly, a study conducted by anthropologist Joseph Dumit (2003) examines the role of brain images experienced by people suffering from mental illness. Dumit describes how brain images potentially alter people's understanding of what he calls their "objective self". The objective self consists of "our taken-for-granted notions, theories, and tendencies regarding human bodies, brains, and kinds considered as objective, referential, extrinsic, and objects of science and medicine" (p. 39). Inspired by Wittgenstein's idea about the production of certainty, Dumit demonstrates how certainty about the brain as the locus of mental illness is produced. Confronted with scientific images of the brain on a daily basis, people become increasingly convinced that these images can tell us who we are. Knowing that we have a brain and that the brain is necessary for our self is therefore a central aspect of our objective self (p. 38).

ADHD is illustrative for how we have come to think about human behaviour as shaped by neurological processes. As I outlined in Chapter 2, understanding of inattention and hyperactivity has changed throughout the past couple of centuries, but the neurobiological explanation has roots in the very early descriptions of children's disruptive behaviour. Even if no biomarkers or brain scanning reveal ADHD, the biologization of ADHD is widely accepted, and as noted by Jutel (2011) and Conrad (2007) among others, patient organizations intensively advocate for the neuro-biological explanation of the disorder. In Chapter 5, I will illustrate how understanding ADHD as a neurobiological disorder opens up a number of interpretations and ways of relating to the diagnosis. The neurobiological explanation forms what Rose calls the register for people diagnosed with ADHD to understand, speak, and act upon themselves, and in Chapter 5 I analyse how the pharmaceutical imaginary, in Jenkins' words, affects the pharmaceutical self. Neither diagnosis nor the explanation of it are neutral. They affect the way we think about ourselves, our possibilities in life, and the constraints we live with.

Concluding remarks

As illustrated in this chapter, we have increasingly come to think of ourselves in diagnostic terms. Psychiatric diagnoses are constructions or selected symptoms clustered together in order to differentiate between different kinds of suffering and coordinate treatment accordingly. Nonetheless, we often think of diagnoses as existing in themselves, independent of the individual's history and the social circumstances in which the individual suffers. We tend to forget that diagnoses change over time and that they have become much more than the clinician's tool for directing treatment. Diagnoses give access to resources and are central for people's organization and request for legitimization of their experienced problems, and in that sense, diagnoses become powerful tools in a fight of social rights. Moreover, diagnoses rearrange identity by offering a specific narrative and grouping the individual with others suffering the same. As the chapter demonstrate, the way we explain and think of diagnoses affects expectations of how to react to suffering and decisions of treatment. These explanations are therefore immensely powerful.

The degree to which we have become neurochemical selves and the question of how or if neurobiology has changed the way we think of the human and of human suffering is debated. Rose (2003) is criticized for overstretching the argument about people exclusively understanding themselves in terms of neurobiology, and critics claim that psychological and social explanations for suffering exist parallel to the neurobiological explanations (Bröer & Heerings, 2013; O'Connor & Joffe, 2013). Rose and Abi-Rached (2013), however, emphasize that personhood is not replaced by "brainhood", but rather that we witness a new register or dimension of selfhood existing alongside other conceptions of personhood. It is, however, clear that neuroscience influences our perception of self, and it is widely acknowledged that we increasingly understand ourselves in neurobiological terms. The implication for each individual may vary, and a relevant question therefore concerns how neurobiological knowledge influences individuals in different situations in life and under different circumstances.

Acknowledgement

This chapter draws on work published in Nielsen, M. (2016). *Experiences of ADHD in adults: Morality, temporality and neurobiology.* Aalborg, Denmark: Aalborg Universitetsforlag. Reprinted by permission of Aalborg Universitetsforlag.

Note

1 For a comparison of different diagnostic practices worldwide see Hinshaw and Scheffler (2014).

References

American Psychiatric Association (APA). (2013). *Diagnostic and statistical manual of mental disorders: DSM-5*. Washington, DC: American Psychiatric Association.

Arnfred, J., & Langager, S. (2015). Diagnoser i Skolen – Elevkarakteristikker og Inklusionspolitikker. In S. Brinkmann & A. Petersen (Eds.), *Diagnoser: Perspektiver, Kritik og Diskussion*. Aarhus, Denmark: Klim.

Barkley, R. A., Murphy, K. R., & Fischer, M. (2008). *ADHD in adults: What the science says*. London: Guilford Press.

Bowker, G. C., & Star, S. L. (2000). *Sorting things out: Classification and its consequences*. Cambridge, MA: MIT Press.

Brinkmann, S. (2014). Psychiatric diagnoses as semiotic mediators: The case of ADHD. *Nordic Psychology*, *66*(2), 121–134.

Brinkmann, S. (2016). *Diagnostic cultures: A cultural approach to the pathologization of modern life*. London: Routledge.

Brinkmann, S., Petersen, A, Kofod, E. H., & Birk, R. (2014). Diagnosekultur: Et Analytisk Perspektiv på Psykiatriske Diagnoser i Samtiden. *Tidsskrift for Norsk Psykologforening*, *51*, 692–697.

Bröer, C., & Heerings, M. (2013). Neurobiology in public and private discourse: The case of adults with ADHD. *Sociology of Health & Illness*, *35*(1), 49–65.

Clarke, A. E., Mamo, L. Fosket, J. R., Fishman, J. R., & Shim, J. K. (2010). *Biomedicalization: Technoscience, health, and illness in the U.S.* Durham, NC and London: Duke University Press.

Conrad, P. (2007). *The medicalization of society: On the transformation of human conditions into treatable disorders*. Baltimore, MD: Johns Hopkins University Press.

Danforth, S., & Navarro, V. (2001). Hyper talk: Sampling the social construction of ADHD in everyday language. *Anthropology & Education Quarterly*, *32*(2), 167–190.

Dumit, J. (2003). Is it me or my brain? Depression and neuroscientific facts. *Journal of Medical Humanities*, *24*(1/2), 35–47.

Farah, M. J. (2012). Neuroethics: The ethical, legal, and societal impact of neuroscience. *Annual Review of Psychology*, *63*(1), 571–591.

Goffman, E. (1959). The moral career of the mental patient. *Psychiatry*, *22*(2), 123–142.

Healy, D. (2012). *Pharmageddon*. Berkeley: University of California Press.

Hinshaw, S. P., & Scheffler, R. M. (2014). *The ADHD explosion: Myths, money, and today's push for performance*. New York, NY: Oxford University Press.

Horton-Salway, M. (2011). Repertoires of ADHD in UK newspaper media. *Health*, *15*(5), 533–549.

Horwitz, A. V. (2002). *Creating mental illness*. Chicago, IL and London: University of Chicago Press.

Illes, J., & Racine, E. (2005). Imaging or imagining? A neuroethics challenge informed by genetics. *American Journal of Bioethics*, *9*(2), 5–18.

Jenkins, J. H. (2010). Psychopharmaceutical self and imaginary in the social field of psychiatric treatment. In J. H Jenkins (Ed.), *Pharmaceutical self: The global shaping of experience in and age of psychopharmacology* (pp. 17–40). Santa Fe, NM: School for Advanced Research.

Jutel, A. (2011). *Putting a name to it*. Baltimore, MD: John Hopkins University Press.

Kleinman, A., & Kleinman, J. (1991). Suffering and its professional transformation: Toward an ethnography of interpersonal experience. *Culture, Medicine and Psychiatry, 15*(3), 275–301.

Kofod, E. H. (2017). From morality to pathology: A brief historization of contemporary Western grief practices and understandings. *Nordic Psychology, 69*(1), 47–60.

Lynch, Z. (2009). *The neuro revolution: How brain science is changing our world.* New York, NY: St. Martin's Press.

Madsen, K. B., Ersbøll, A. K., Olsen, J., Parner, E., & Obel, C. (2015). Geographic analysis of the variation in the incidence of ADHD in a country with free access to health care: A Danish cohort study. *International Journal of Health Geographics, 14*(1), 1–13.

Martin, E. (2007). *Bipolar expeditions: Mania and depression in American culture.* Oxford: Princeton University Press.

Mayes, R., & Horwitz, A. V. (2005). DSM-III and the revolution in the classification of mental illness. *Journal of the History of Behavioral Sciences, 4*(3), 249–267.

Mirowsky, J., & Ross, C. E. (1989). Psychiatric diagnosis as reified measurement. *Journal of Health and Social Behavior, 30*(1), 11–25.

Mol, A. (2002). *The body multiple: Ontology in medical practice.* Durham, NC: Duke University Press.

O'Connor, C., & Joffe, H. (2013). How has neuroscience affected lay understandings of personhood? A review of the evidence. *Public Understanding of Science, 22*(3), 254–268.

Rose, N. (2003). Neurochemical selves. *Society, 41*(1), 46–59.

Rose, N. (2006). Disorders without borders? The expanding scope of psychiatric practice. *BioSocieties, 1*, 465–484.

Rose, N. (2013). What is diagnosis for? Talk given at the Institute of Psychiatry, King's College, London.

Rose, N., & Abi-Rached, J. M. (2013). *Neuro: The new brain sciences and the management of the mind.* Princeton, NJ: Princeton University Press.

Novas, C., & Rose, N. (2000). Genetic risk and the birth of the somatic individual. *Economy and Society, 29*(4), 485–513.

Rosenberg, C. E. (2002). The tyranny of diagnosis: Specific entities and individual experience. *Milbank Quarterly, 80*(2), 237–260.

Rosenberg, C. E. (2006). Contested boundaries: Psychiatry, disease, and diagnosis. *Perspectives in Biology and Medicine, 49*(3), 407–424.

Scheper-Hughes, N., & Lock, M. (1987). The mindful body: A prolegomenon to future work in medical anthropology. *Medical Anthropology Quarterly, 1*, 6–41.

Singh, I., & Rose, N. (2006). Neuro-forum: An introduction. *BioSocieties, 1*(1), 97–102.

Sundhedsstyrelsen. (2015). *National klinisk retningslinje for udredning og behandling af ADHD hos voksne – med forstyrrelse af aktivitet og opmærksomhed samt opmærksomhedsforstyrrelse uden hyperaktivitet.* København, Denmark: Sundhedsstyrelsen.

Wallach-Kildemoes, H. M., Skovgaard, A. H., Thielen, K., Pottegård, A., & Mortensen, L. (2015). Social adversity and regional differences in prescribing of ADHD medication for school-age children. *Journal of Developmental & Behavioral Pediatrics, 36*(5), 330–341.

Whitaker, R. (2010). *Anatomy of an epidemic: Magic bullets, psychiatric drugs, and the astonishing rise of mental illness in America.* New York, NY: Broadway Books.

World Health Organization (WHO). (2018). *International statistical classification of diseases and related health problems* (11th revision). Retrieved from https://icd.who.int/browse11/l-m/en.

Chapter 4

Experiences and implications of getting an ADHD diagnosis

It is a readjustment process relating to it [the diagnosis]. For a period of time, I was looking at my life through ADHD glasses before I was able to separate things from each other. I mean: what [in me] was ADHD? All the things in my life. What if I did not have ADHD? All of a sudden you reconsider a lot of things and think: what could have happened [if I did not have ADHD] and how? It was a process I had to go through. But those first months – when you had to find out what exactly it meant – they were tough.

(Louise, 26 years old, diagnosed with ADHD
three years prior to the interview)

How can we understand experiences of getting an ADHD diagnosis and the social, practical, and moral implications and considerations that follow? And what does the diagnosis tell us about who we are and who we can become? Early in my fieldwork, I met Louise for an interview. Louise is a student, she lives with her boyfriend, and is being treated with a central nervous stimulant for ADHD. Louise has dropped out of high school three times but is currently in the midst of her studies again. The first two times she had to leave her studies was because she struggled with all the demands in school. The third time was because she was diagnosed with and treated for depression. As part of the treatment, Louise was asked to write down her life story, about her childhood, her family, her experiences at school, and the different twists and turns her life has taken. Identifying symptoms of ADHD in Louise's story, her doctor passed on her writings to a psychiatrist, however this was done without letting Louise know of his suspicions. Louise was therefore utterly surprised when confronted with the psychiatrist's evaluation that she might have ADHD. Louise recalls: "I was so confused. I thought we were going to talk about depression – and now he mentions ADHD." Louise knew very little about ADHD and could not see herself fitting into her conception of someone with ADHD. "That is for little boys," she thought. But the more the psychiatrist explained about ADHD, the more Louise recognized herself in the diagnostic descriptions. And when her mother was invited to the psychiatrist's office for an interview about Louise's childhood, they both realized that Louise has always struggled with symptoms of ADHD.

Louise's story indicates how new ways of being, acting, and understanding oneself often accompany a diagnosis. Louise wonders what ADHD is, how her life is affected by it, and how to understand her everyday struggles in the light of the diagnosis. Her ambiguous and open-ended questions represent some of the speculations and thoughts of evaluation that often follow during and after a diagnostic process. Louise is about to learn how to live with and manage symptoms of ADHD. How to structure everyday tasks, take medication, and deal with others' reactions to the diagnosis. The diagnosis and the following treatment have helped Louise in many respects – to such a degree that she and her family differentiate between the "before-Louise" and the "after-Louise". She told me that, "The life I lived before and the life I live now, it is really not the same. Not at all."

As I have shown in the previous chapters, psychiatric diagnoses have been heavily criticized for being stigmatizing, over-inclusive, and pathologizing (Conrad, 2007; Horwitz, 2002), and the critical contributions to the debate over the medicalization of society are valuable. What these studies do not examine, however, is the individual's experience of being diagnosed and the consequences of living with, learning from, and being restricted by a diagnosis. In this chapter, I examine experiences of getting an ADHD diagnosis in adulthood and the implications following the diagnosis – some directly caused by the effect of medication, some by the explanatory force of the diagnosis, and others by the careful crafting of new practices. As noted in Chapter 3, anamnesis must demonstrate symptoms of ADHD from the age of 12 or earlier in order to be diagnosed with ADHD. Hence, a diagnosis in adulthood offers a framework for interpretation that captures a whole life's sensations, feelings, and patterns of behaviour. The diagnosis answers a number of questions and helps the diagnosed to identify, accept, and cope with problems by offering concrete explanations and treatment for the problems experienced. However, even if the diagnosis is a great help for many, the diagnostic process is not only illuminating but also brings new challenges and questions. Relating to the diagnosis and testing drugs is a process full of experiments and readjustments, in which the individual must turn their attention inwards and evaluate everyday problems (Nielsen, 2018). Therefore, acquiring and making use of the diagnosis happens in all sorts of settings and everyday practices.

Through excerpts from my fieldwork, I demonstrate how getting an ADHD diagnosis is a process in which existential questions are raised and everyday practices are scrutinized, evaluated, and often changed. I illustrate how the diagnostic process entails a process of recognizing oneself as someone with ADHD, crafting new skills, and continuous self-evaluations and moral considerations. My interlocutors describe their life as chaotic, their thoughts as messy, and they report of a life full of misunderstandings and of always feeling "different". In their struggle to find calmness in life, the diagnosis is helpful. It helps order chaos in different ways by structuring self-understandings, giving new guidelines for practices, and changing experiences and perceptions through medication. As I will show in this chapter, the process of being diagnosed with ADHD often entails several months or even years of exploring the possibilities and limitations of the diagnosis.

The explanatory force of a diagnosis and questions of responsibility

Getting a diagnosis is in many ways like getting a verdict. A verdict that demarcates the normal from the abnormal, health from pathology, and that places responsibility. The process of examining and completing anamnesis, scrutinizing childhood behaviour, school performance, and social skills as part of a diagnostic process could be seen to symbolically parallel the justi-fication and confession of the courtroom, where the individual is the object of study. They are pointed at as the locus of the problem and are expected to take the necessary measures: to acknowledge the verdict and manage what led to the verdict. But even if a diagnosis shares some of the same features as a verdict, a diagnosis does not work like a verdict. Contrary to the verdict in courtrooms, verdicts in the clinic are often appreciated, and the people I have talked to as part of my fieldwork welcomed the diagnosis and accepted it as a long-awaited explanation for their problems. Ambiguous mechanisms are at play during a diagnostic process, and acceptance of the diagnosis is partly understood by noticing how responsibility is both installed in and taken away from the individual. On the one hand, the investigated problem is located within the individual rather than in the individual's surroundings, and the individual is thereby held responsible for changing what is considered prob-lematic. But on the other hand, the problem is translated from a personal flaw into a diagnosis, which thereby relieves the individual from responsibility. A shift from morally to medically evaluating behavioural problems therefore transforms the status of the judgement (Conrad, 2007).

In the following, one of my interlocutors, whom I call John, describes how the diagnosis changed his ideas about himself and his problems. Concentration was never John's strong point, and during his bachelor-degree studies, he realized that he needed help to focus. The assignments seemed unmanageable and John felt stupid and useless. Searching for help, he contacted a hypno-therapist to adjust and straighten out his disorganized thoughts and was therefore quite surprised to hear that the therapist suspected his inability to concentrate to be symptoms of ADHD. Never had he suspected that himself. But on the therapist's friendly request, he went to see a psychiatrist, who eventually diagnosed him with ADHD. While the diagnosis was a surprise, John also remembers the relief he felt when finally getting an explanation for his struggles. As a culmination of feeling different for years, followed by months of assessing and weighing symptoms, the diagnosis offered him a new perspective. John explains:

> It is because you think you're wrong or something. That is how I felt [before the diagnosis]. There must be something wrong with me. I might be stupid or something. And then you get that: it is ADHD. And then you think: okay, then there is a reason for me to be the way I am.

During my fieldwork, my interlocutors continuously told me that the diagnosis offered an explanation to a life full of difficulties. Throughout their lives, they have experienced negative judgements from family members, teachers, and friends, and reviewing the past as problematic and full of failure was a common characterization. Just as John has always thought of his difficulties as a consequence of him being stupid, so have others interpreted his problems. The diagnosis therefore not only legitimizes difficulties in terms of reducing self-blame, it also serves as an explanation in conversation with others.

Kenny, whom I met later during my fieldwork, also characterizes the time he was diagnosed as a turning point in life. Explaining about his family's reaction to the diagnosis, Kenny, describes his father's devastation over not being able to interpret his son's problems as symptoms of ADHD. Kenny was diagnosed at the age of 30, after learning about the condition as part of his studies and subsequently asking his doctor for a diagnostic examination. Generally, Kenny considers his childhood as being happy, but he also remembers controversies, corrections, and reprimands when the clashes in communication between him and his father escalated. That, however has now changed. Kenny recollects his father's reaction to the diagnosis:

> He [the father] completely broke down. [He said,] "We have treated you wrong your whole life" and things like that. Because I was bawled out a lot as a kid. And, "Why the hell was I not able to behave and align?" I mean, they felt powerless. "Why can you not just be like everybody else?" In that kind of way. But now he suddenly realized that I could not help it and I was not doing things on purpose. It was just the way I was.

The diagnosis makes it possible to account for previous conflicts and controversies to family and friends using a legitimate explanation, just as it enables conversations about previous problems within a very specific and confined framework that allows for tolerance and forgiveness. Kenny experienced a reconciliation with his farther after finally being able to talk about his own problems as well as their family dynamics from a new perspective. A perspective that changed interpretations of responsibility and rearranged responsibilities. While Kenny is relieved from responsibility for his actions, his father experiences a new kind of guilt for not being able to understand his son's behaviour correctly and not providing the necessary support and guidance. The diagnosis therefore rearranges not only Kenny's perception of himself but also has extensive implications on how Kenny and his family members think of themselves as a family.

Restructuring narratives and self-perceptions

An ADHD diagnosis often enters people's lives during an evaluative moment in life when problems have become insurmountable and questions about the nature of these problems require answers. During such a turbulent time, the process of being diagnosed contributes to the evaluation process with its interrogation of childhood habits and everyday actions. Charts and questionnaires are filled out, and for each box with symptoms ticked off in a test, a pattern of behaviour is slowly transferred into a diagnosis. Ann, who was diagnosed half a year before I interviewed her, tells me how the past year had brought about various changes as she got divorced and was diagnosed with whiplash after a car accident. Throughout her life, Ann has tried to manage her problems, yet repeatedly experienced failure. Ann and her family have a history of various psychological problems (Ann was a cutter for years), and in this light, the ADHD diagnosis encapsulates a culmination of a life full of difficulties and obstacles. The diagnosis enters into a process of readjustments and contributes to the clarification of thoughts and life choices. It directs Ann forward by offering explanations and treatment for her problems. Ann describes her reaction to the diagnosis:

> Well, it [the diagnosis] made me realize why I struggle with some things. Before, I never got a hold on why I was struggling and why I was the way I was. [I] was so stressed out when too many things were happening. I kind of have a different understanding now, and I know how to act more appropriately. Things have got – well it has not eliminated the problems – but it [the diagnosis] has given me an insight into why these problems occur. It made it possible for me to pin up my reactions and challenges to something. And in that way, I am actually happy and relieved to finally discover what was troubling me. I believe [that since the diagnosis] I am nicer and kinder to myself.

The diagnosis offers a clear and concrete vocabulary to speak about experiences that can otherwise be difficult to verbalize. It systematizes experiences of continuously bumping into problems and conflicts, and the list of symptoms and descriptions of typical problems related to ADHD gives clarity to what were previously diffuse challenges. The diagnosis becomes what Brinkmann (2014) calls a semiotic mediator for individuals to use in order "to understand and act toward their moods, emotions, thoughts, actions, and problems" (p. 123). Thus, the diagnosis becomes a tool for ordering life, understanding one's differentness, and working on how to cope with it. Similarly, Ann describes how she experienced a sense of relief because the diagnosis provided the opportunity for thinking differently about herself.

As outlined in Chapter 3, a diagnosis transforms unorganized illness experiences and suffering into a rationalized and organized disorder (Conrad & Potter, 2000). The diagnosis in effect collects scattered experiences and connects them into an entity and a treatable condition. This function of bringing clarity and structure is described by Jutel (2011) as follows:

> Receiving a diagnosis is like being handed a road map in the middle of a forest. It shows the way – but not necessarily the way out. It indicates what the path ahead is going to look like, where it will lead, the difficulty of the climb, and various potential turn-offs along the way. Perhaps it identifies a destination, but not necessarily. With a diagnosis, things not necessarily get better, but they become clearer. The unexplained becomes explained, and management is defined. Assumptions are made about the future.
>
> (p. 1)

If we return to Ann, we can understand Ann's descriptions of being diagnosed as being handed a map. From the point of view of a tangible, well-described disorder, indicating specific difficulties and offering certain guidelines, Ann's problems are easier to address. The diagnosis might not eliminate problems, but it makes them clearer. After being diagnosed, Ann changed her perception of herself. She interprets her history in the light of the diagnosis and uses the diagnosis to explain her actions and her confused and troubled life. With the diagnosis in hand, Ann gives herself a new history. A history that centres around ADHD and outlines how symptoms of ADHD have been crucial for how things in her life have developed. Rosenberg (2002) notes that diagnosing is "a ritual of disclosure", when "a curtain is pulled aside, and uncertainty is replaced – for better or for worse – by a structured narrative" (p. 255). Ann experiences that the diagnosis transforms her experiences into a story of difficulties that has a certain structure and that she shares with others diagnosed with ADHD. ADHD becomes a category that recapitulates the individual's experiences and the diagnosis is used as the knot that binds together the past, the present, and future possibilities. The diagnosis is based upon the individual's life story, but at the same time it offers a specific vocabulary and narrative framework for the individual to interpret their life through. In this way, to get an ADHD diagnosis is a process of reconstructing self-perceptions as focus shifts from an unfounded differentness and sense of failure to an understanding of behaviour that is evidence of a diagnosis.

Evaluating yourself and considering new questions

We often tend to think of a diagnosis as a category given to an individual at a certain time and place. But getting a diagnosis is not just a single event. A whole life's experiences and sometimes a long diagnostic process lies behind it and even if the individual is relieved to get the diagnosis as an explanation to their challenges, the time after officially getting the diagnosis is often accompanied with questions of doubt and considerations relating to the diagnosis. The diagnosis answers questions and offers explanations for the individual's suffering, but it also raises a number of questions during the diagnostic process as well as after the diagnosis is assigned. From the moment the individual is given the diagnosis, a process of assessing and evaluating the person's reactions and behavioural patterns begins, and as no biological tests can determine if you have ADHD, the diagnosis is based on an analysis of the individual's life story and description of their experienced problems. Being able to identify and verbalize experiences is therefore a pre-requisite for the psychiatrist to be able to accurately diagnose. But identifying and verbalizing bodily sensations and difficulties in life is not always an easy task.

During my fieldwork I visited Patricia and Peter. Peter got his diagnosis at the age of 25, after a time of stress and symptoms of depression. Peter particularly remembers one day that he vomited from feeling overwhelmingly stressed out, and Patricia insisted he acknowledged his problems and went to see a therapist. And so he did. While sitting on the couch with Peter and talking about the dramatic time when he was diagnosed, I ask about the diagnostic process and how the diagnosis was determined. Peter tells me that he was handed a form with questions about everyday habits and boxes indicating different degrees of problematic behaviour. Peter and Patricia were asked to fill out the form together, which, it turned out, was not an easy task. Despite sharing their everyday life together, coming more or less to terms with Peter's difficulties, they did not agree on how to answer the questionnaire. In the following, Patricia and Peter outline why:

PATRICIA: Well he could not see that there was anything wrong. It [the behaviour described in the questionnaire] is just how he is.

PETER: To me it is normal. The things described in the form were just things I normally do. I do not even remember what it said.

PATRICIA: But you do not know how to listen to yourself and your body, so to be able to see yourself from the outside that does not really work with you. Not until I explained it to you: "When you do it like that or like that" – I could give you tons of examples … then you realized – what you assessed to be "mild degrees: were maybe to be located at the other end of the scale. So, it took some time to fill out the form.

AUTHOR: So, when you say you ticked the box indicating "mild degree" it was because you thought everybody feels this way? You did not think of it as something special?

PETER: Not at all. I thought it was normal. Well it was not, I realized.

To fill out the questionnaire requires an ability to pay attention to your body, reflect over your everyday life and routines, and assess your own reactions and behaviour. Peter finds those exercises difficult. His family is unfamiliar with talking about personal problems, Peter and Patricia agree that they have never really targeted Peter's life-long experiences of restlessness. To analyse himself is therefore something he is unaccustomed to and his difficulty in ticking off the boxes raises the question, how is it possible to judge if the way your feel and react is normal? Normal to Peter is how he has always perceived himself and the world around him. He acknowledges that he has some problems that need to be dealt with, but to determine the level of, for example, forgetting appointments or interrupting others is an intricate affair. Along the same line, Karen, whom we met in the beginning of this book, describes the paradox of assessing yourself during the diagnostic process based on an ideal of the normal or the common. In her case, however, it was the psychiatrist, and not the diagnostic questionnaire, who asked her to depict her differentness. Karen explains:

I have moved around quite a lot. And I have had relatively many relationships. I had all the classic characteristics. But when I have to describe myself, how I deviate from someone normal, how should I be able to do that? I know what is normal to me, but I do not know what is normal to you or to the average person. I could not do that. And that is why I could not put it into words.

While the diagnosis may offer a vocabulary that gives concrete expression to diffuse experiences (and thereby makes it possible to describe your differences to others) you must be able to evaluate yourself, look at yourself from the gaze of an outsider, and pinpoint your problems in order to access this resource. The process of getting a diagnosis is therefore rather demanding in terms of skills of self-evaluation and verbal expression.

It is not only the diagnostic examination that raises new questions. The process after being diagnosed also leaves the individual in a state of grappling with the implications of being diagnosed. As Louise says in the beginning of this chapter, suddenly you have to understand yourself through a set of ADHD glasses. You have to accommodate to a new system with its own logic and language in order for the diagnosis to make sense. The diagnosis activates new kinds of reflections – especially to those who never thought of their difficulties as symptoms of ADHD. Neither Louise nor John suspected ADHD before they went through a diagnostic examination. Accepting and understanding the implications of being diagnosed therefore took a while. In the following, John describes his sense of confusion after being diagnosed:

> So, I just stood there. I knew nothing about ADHD whatsoever. I had to go online and figure out my possibilities. I am kind of still doing that, because there is not much information to get. You are like thrown into a labyrinth, and you do not know your way to begin with. That was my reaction to the diagnosis. It was a weird thing to get that diagnosis, I think.

The relief of getting a diagnosis is sometimes followed by a process of exploring the consequences of being diagnosed. Returning to the quote by Jutel (2011) about the diagnosis being a map without any indication of locality, John's description of being thrown into a labyrinth expresses a similar metaphorical picture of the diagnosis as a system, a meaningful instrument, which you as the diagnosed must learn to navigate and master. The diagnosis may have a powerful explanatory force, but being able to profit from it, requires a reasonable amount of effort.

Restructuring practices and crafting skills

After being diagnosed, certain tasks lie ahead. The person diagnosed must relate to the diagnosis, include it in his or her life story, and act upon it in order to address the identified problems. In other words, the diagnosis renders new ways of being and acting possible. Ann explains how the diagnosis makes her "know how to act more appropriately" when problems occur. She is, for example, more aware of organizing her daily activities such as choosing the right time of day for grocery shopping, in order to avoid being overstimulated by the presence of other people during rush hours. Knowing how to react more appropriately, however, also involves reflections over how to manage one's mood and temper. Thus, the diagnosis not only explains past events and current problems, it also offers prospects for the future and new ways of thinking about responsibility.

After John was diagnosed with ADHD, he was unsure how to benefit from the diagnosis – even if he believed it correctly characterized his problems. The medication had too many negative side effects, and John realized that he had to cope with the symptoms of ADHD differently. Looking back at the process, John remembers feeling lost for a while, struggling to find his way around the diagnosis. His psychiatrist was more preoccupied with testing medication, John recollects, and less interested in talking about John's reflections about being diagnosed and the consequences of living with ADHD. So he had to find out himself. Today, John believes the diagnosis has been significant in his search for a way of dealing with his problems. "I am better at some things now knowing that I have ADHD and knowing that there are some tools for managing it," John says. The diagnosis made him curious to learn about and cope with his difficulties and not only has he started reading about ADHD, he has even started attending a self-financed ADHD coaching course in order to learn about the condition further. As a result of the course, John is practising new techniques for coping with his temper and impulsivity and in the following John answers my question about how these practices work:

> Well, it is all about training the brain, and about training myself to do things differently. To notice when the habitual behaviour comes. And then stop it and say: all right let us go this way instead. I mean, when you react to something, you react based on feelings. And then you need to notice: When do these feelings come? When am I getting angry? What happened? Take a step back and notice: When am I getting angry? What is the reason? What were my feelings before I got angry? And then next time [I] notice that feeling, instead of getting angry, I will try to take it easy. Like that … it does not just happen like that … I think you need to practice for some years. Multiple times.

According to John, the diagnosis has become a tool for changing his way of thinking and acting. He does not always succeed in incorporating the techniques from the coaching course, but he is continuously testing, examining, and crafting new skills and learning how to control what he now identifies as ADHD behaviour. While the diagnosis is determined in the psychiatrist's office, the practice of relating to it, discovering what it entails, and how to benefit from it happens in all sorts of places and is a long process that demands the incorporation of new routines and continuous practice.

As Petersen and Madsen (2017) argue, "Getting, living with and ascribing meaning to the diagnosis" (p. 25) is a process. Different kinds of treatment often follow the diagnosis and new practices and ways of administrating everyday tasks are refined in the effort of managing what is now defined and characterized as ADHD.

Just as John uses the diagnosis as a tool for changing some inexpedient thinking and behavioural patterns, Karen describes the process after being diagnosed as a time in life when she started developing new strategies. But contrary to John's experiences, medication has played a significant role for Karen. She has always been very energetic and struggled to maintain focus. Medication, however, enabled her to find calmness. Karen explains:

> When I got the ADHD diagnosis, I became calm. The reason I became calm was because I got medication. And that enabled me to suddenly start understanding myself. I started using my strengths in a more focused way, I found a kind of balance, and I started developing new strategies. I have always had many strategies for how to live life.

Living with undiagnosed ADHD, Karen had always been a master of developing strategies in order to fit in, and getting the diagnosis became yet another strategy for her to manage the recurrent problems. Just like John, Karen and my other interlocutors make use of the diagnosis and the resources following it when trying to manage their problems in life. Everyday practices are redefined in the effort towards "living in chaos and striving for control" (Toner, O'Donoghue, & Houghton, 2006, p. 247). During my fieldwork, I have encountered several practices related to the cultivation of new strategies to manage behaviour after the diagnosis. In ADHD-related online forums, people ask for advice in order to gain control in a chaotic life. And while some, like John, choose to attend courses that offers ADHD management strategies, others experiment with strategies for gaining control. A couple of home visits during my fieldwork illustrate two specific practices of trying to manage difficulties related to ADHD:

One autumn afternoon, I visit Kelly, a 26-year-old woman diagnosed with ADHD a couple of years before our meeting. She tells me that her reaction when introduced to ADHD was, "Well, just another box for me to fit into". She was previously diagnosed with dyslexia only to be deprived of that diagnosis later. To be put in another box, therefore, did not impress Kelly at first. However, learning more about the diagnosis and being helped by medical treatment, Kelly is now convinced the diagnosis is correct. She now strongly identifies with it, she tells me, while we sit at the dining table. In the adjoining room, I discover a big white board and Kelly explains that she uses the board as her external memory. Repeatedly, she and her boyfriend argue about daily planning: who said what, when to do what, and structuring each day and each activity by plotting it on the white board helps Kelly navigate. Kelly tells me that her working memory is impaired – or that her ability to remember things might be affected by the fact that she gets very easily distracted as part of her ADHD. Incorporating the white board as a structuring element keeps her focused and able to perform everyday tasks. Every activity is (supposed) to appear on the white board for Kelly to remember to do it and for the written word to communicate between Kelly and her boyfriend. Paradoxically, dividing each day into separate activities – by splitting it into different fragments – establishes continuity in her life and a kind of maintenance in her easily distracted mind.

When I visit another of my interlocutors, Evelyn, her strategy for structuring daily routines reminds me of Kelly's description of the white board as her external memory. Evelyn is in her mid-forties and is going through a turbulent time. Like herself, her adult son has just been diagnosed with ADHD and she is determined to start a new chapter in life with more stability and care for herself. Evelyn tells me that her biggest problem related to ADHD is her inability to maintain a structured life. Her handbag is a mess, her apartment is a mess, and her life has somehow always been messy. But the ADHD diagnosis and the following treatment have helped her find some kind of order in her chaotic life, she tells me, showing me a picture of her messy apartment just a few months ago. Besides her medical treatment, the municipality has offered her a body awareness therapy course and a mentor who helps her clean up the apartment, which she describes as essential in enabling her to take action in her life. As part of the treatment plan, she has made her own system of boxes, bags, and hooks for her to remember where she puts her stuff. She points at her wall and desk where all sorts of coloured boxes store make-up, keys, pencils, notebooks, etc. Like a large- scale printer's drawer, the rear end of Evelyn's apartment keeps most of the things she needs from the moment she wakes up until she leaves in the morning. The installations make me think of an external brain, in which different areas hold different functions: a tangible, practical memory system that visually communicates what needs to be done during the day. Some things are for morning rituals, others are for studying, and together the installation materializes the ordering of everyday practices. These small installations come forward – they somehow illustrate and orchestrate their own purpose – and they become part of Evelyn's way of acting and thinking. A combination of medical treatment and practical help in housekeeping has enabled Evelyn to incorporate new practices and ways of handling her difficulty with structure. She still sometimes forgets things, but she carefully uses new techniques and crafts new skills in order to function better.

Like every person diagnosed with ADHD I have talked to, Evelyn is exploring how she is affected by symptoms of ADHD and is facing her difficulties. She is determined to overcome her problems and is exerting all her energy into the art of crafting herself as a person who is able to navigate in ordered chaos. This practice is a continuous challenge of self-evaluation that demands repetitive exercise before it is incorporated into everyday life. As I will describe further in Chapter 5, in a world of structure, with certain ways of organizing and certain rhythms in life, each person is impelled to make use of the available means in order to adapt to normative demands of leading an ordered life. An ADHD diagnosis can be such a means, whether it be the explanatory force of it, the prescription of drugs, or the guidelines for being aware of and changing behavioural patterns, to help the diagnosed further in this process. Getting the diagnosis is a readjustment process, and it is an opportunity for "stepping back and trying to look at myself, observe myself … my unfavourable features, and what do I do about it", as Christian, a man diagnosed four years before I met him, puts it. Knowledge about ADHD becomes an integrated part of new as well as existing strategies, and learning to live with and manage symptoms of ADHD is a process of continuously restructuring everyday practices. A diagnosis may give access to resources, as described in Chapter 3, but the majority of the workload rests with the individual and their to benefit from the diagnosis.

Ambivalence towards the diagnosis

Sociological studies of psychiatric diagnoses and consequences of being diagnosed often point to the harsh stigma attached to these kinds of categorizations (Goffman, 1963). Contrary to somatic diagnoses, psychiatric diagnoses are connected to moral blame and social exclusion, and studies of ADHD reveal that people diagnosed with ADHD keep the diagnosis to themselves due to fear of stigmatization (Young, Bramham, Gray, & Rose, 2008). Some even reject the diagnosis and feel misrepresented by it.[1] During my fieldwork, I met people with different feelings of ambivalence towards the diagnosis, even if everyone accepted it. Concerns about the legal aspects of being diagnosed with ADHD were also shared among my interlocutors and some of them worry if authorities will judge them by the diagnosis and treat them differently, resulting in difficulties with employment, insurance, and generally maintaining equal rights after the diagnosis. For example, one of my interlocutors was asked to try medication when officially evaluated for income support. Another considered if he should add to his job applications that he was diagnosed with ADHD. And yet another was in the middle of a legal fight about whether or not she was obliged to inform her employer about the diagnosis before she started her new job. Generally, however, ambivalence towards the diagnosis were often connected to aspects about coming to terms with being perceived as someone with ADHD. Besides using knowledge about the disorder to positively reconstruct self-perceptions, some experience doubts and conflicting thoughts following the diagnosis. The people I have talked to are aware that ADHD is a controversial diagnosis and they struggle to position themselves as legitimately diagnosed. At the same time, they have to fight others' narrow conception of what ADHD is and their stereotypical ideas of who a person with ADHD is. As discussed in Chapter 3, the legitimacy of the diagnosis relies on whether it corresponds with what is recognized as a valid explanation and whether the patient accepts the narrative offered by the diagnosis. In order for the diagnosis to make sense, the narrative must resonate with the person's self-perception – even it brings about new perspectives and ways of understanding oneself. But the explanatory power of the diagnosis is also dependent on whether others are able to equate the person diagnosed with the diagnosis.

Social representation theories examine how individuals identify with and are being identified with prototypes. According to these theories, a given category of people entails a specific prototype, of which we have certain conceptions. As an example, studies show that the prototype of ADHD is a young, white man or boy (Schmitz, Filippone, & Edelman, 2003). That is how the typical person with ADHD is most likely portrayed and that is how we understand the prototype. This prototype affects who we instinctively diagnose with ADHD because we focus on the patterns of behaviour that fit into the prototype. The prototype also affects how we perceive of people diagnosed with ADHD, and finally it affects the people diagnosed with ADHD and the degree to which they identify with the diagnosis. Sometimes the prototype is hard to identify with and it can take some time to get accustomed to, and sometimes it is necessary to challenge both one's own and others' prejudices about who a person with ADHD is. Especially some of the women I have interviewed have troubles identifying with the stereotypical picture of someone with ADHD: "I'm not a young, restless boy!" In my study, I met three general concerns: that others would not accept the diagnosis to be true, that the diagnosis might cause discrimination, and that narrow ideas about who the person with ADHD is restricted others from seeing the whole person. Kelly had all three concerns and to illustrate these, she explains how fellow students or friends of friends often want to put her "in an ADHD box", whereas at other times, they question her diagnosis:

> I am afraid of being labelled: "Well you are like this because you have ADHD. But you do not live up to having ADHD so you must be lying."

If you do not live up to the precise prejudice people have, it does not make sense [to them]. So being ADHD is living completely up to that stereotype.

While Kelly experiences the ADHD diagnosis as liberating because of its ability to offer explanations for her difficulties, it is also constraining since it offers only a limited set of roles. Being well medicated and slowly learning to cope with her difficulties, Kelly does not resemble the prototypical ADHD person and she does not fit into people's conception of who a person with ADHD is. Therefore, people have a hard time recognizing her as someone with ADHD and they presume she must be one of those subjected to overdiagnosis. Moreover, telling others about her diagnosis, Kelly explains, may also have another unwanted consequence: She has noticed that some people change their behaviour towards her, giving her some kind of, what she perceives to be, positive special treatment, which she certainly does not want. The diagnosis must never be an excuse, as she puts it. Kelly thus constantly tries to manoeuvre in a social landscape where she has to convince others that she is rightly diagnosed with ADHD, and at the same time refuse to be treated differently.

Experiencing the constraints of the diagnosis, Kelly is also afraid the diagnosis will prevent her from achieving things in life. She worries that the diagnosis will turn out be a self-fulfilling prophecy, and that she will eventually be like one of those prototypical images of a person with ADHD. As part of researching about ADHD and trying to figure out what the diagnosis entails, Kelly stumbled upon an online forum for adults diagnosed with the condition. Hoping she would be inspired and be able to share experiences with others, she joined the group, only to quickly leave it again. The conversations were devastating to read, she tells me. Kelly had just started studying when she was diagnosed, but she insisted on finishing her exams. People in the forum, on the contrary, all seemed to be living on benefits from social services, and reading about these stories, knowing that they all shared the same diagnosis, was too discouraging. At the time, Kelly needed to maintain belief in the possibility of a different path in life than the one she was presented to in the forum and even today, she still needs to remind herself that the prototypical ADHD trajectory in life is not necessarily hers. She therefore tries to navigate between, on the one hand, accepting the diagnosis when understanding herself and, on the other hand, insisting on maintaining individual characteristics and being different in her own specific way. As Kelly's story shows, being diagnosed with ADHD does not necessarily mean buying "the whole ADHD package" (Andersen, 2009, p. 122), or accepting the stereotypical roles connected to ADHD.

Research on adults' experiences of being diagnosed with ADHD shows that some adults are afraid the diagnosis will turn into a self-fulfilling prophecy, either because their possibilities in life are underestimated by others or because knowledge about difficulties associated with ADHD can result in loss of self-confidence and lack of courage to explore new possibilities (Halleröd, Anckarsäter, Råstam, & Scherman, 2015). Fearing that the diagnosis will guide one's choices in life and thereby restrain one from doing things considered challenging or impossible for people diagnosed with ADHD, leads to ambivalence towards the diagnosis. As previously described, the diagnosis structures the past, present, and future into a coherent story and thereby also creates prospects for the future. Kelly's story exemplifies the disturbing aspect of seeing a certain trajectory in life associated with a diagnosis and the challenge it is to imagine another life. But Kelly's story also illustrates how discrimination and stigmatization are complex phenomena that not only refer to concerns about the stigma attached to psychiatric diagnoses but also about the legitimacy of the diagnosis and the continuous negotiations about who the ADHD person is and what characteristics and expected behaviour the diagnosis entails. My interlocutors strategically chose who to inform about the diagnosis because of tiresome arguments concerning whether or not they are rightly diagnosed and because of stigma attached to the diagnosis. However, it is important to note that throughout their lives, they have experienced stigma in various degrees because they often deviate from the norm. The ADHD diagnosis is therefore described as generally reducing stigma rather than enforcing it, regardless of whatever discussion might follow regarding the legitimacy of the diagnosis.

Taking medication and experimenting with experiences

Clinical guidelines recommend treatment for ADHD with central nervous system stimulants and during my fieldwork I discovered that for most adults diagnosed with ADHD, testing different substances are part of being diagnosed. Prescription of drugs is a kind of social act or written agreement, in which the doctor recognizes the patient's suffering (Van der Geest, Whyte, & Hardon, 1996). Similarly, I observed that talking about the effect of drugs, evaluating labels of drugs, and readjusting the dosage of drugs is a central aspect of being diagnosed with and treated for ADHD.

One late autumn morning, I follow Peter to his psychiatrist, whom he frequently sees in order to adjust his medication. On the way, Peter tells me that he wants to increase the dosage – he feels like he needs it. In the consultation room, Peter sits on the edge of the chair and seems a bit restless. Together Peter and the psychiatrist enumerate the Motiron pills, a central nervous stimulant, that Peter takes during the day. It appears to be a familiar practice happening automatically. The psychiatrist looks at his computer and Peter looks at the app on his phone, where he keeps track of his medication. The psychiatrist says, "4, 2, 2, 2, 1." "No," Peter corrects him, "4, 2, 2, 3, 2." "In the night, I take two – and then sometimes I take one between 5 pm and 10 pm." The psychiatrist nods and corrects the data on the screen. "Then you are within the normal spectrum," he assures Peter. Peter is very cautious when it comes to his medication. If he messes up the order or time of the pills, he loses focus, becomes irritated, or his sleep is disturbed. Working full-time, keeping the house, and taking care of two kids and a dog requires structure, and Peter is struggling to figure out what combination and types of drugs help to best facilitate this. The dialogue between Peter and his psychiatrist illustrates how communication about dosage becomes a medium for talking about Peter's current state. Medication is an adjustable parameter, and agreeing on an appropriate dosage satisfies both Peter's and the psychiatrist's wish for improving his situation. The situation, however, also illustrates the continuous evaluation and readjustment process of testing the desired state of well-being. In other words, assessing the dosage of drugs is an experiment in discovering the effect that corresponds to the individual's expectations.

As mentioned in previous chapters, medical treatment of ADHD is widely critiqued for being a tool for enhancement rather than for treating genuine disorders (Conrad, 2007; Timimi & Leo, 2009). Despite this, many people diagnosed with ADHD accept and sometimes even welcome medical treatment. Without exception, all of my interlocutors have tried different drugs, and while some experience unwanted side effects and choose to stop treatment, others benefit from it. They all accept treatment with central nervous stimulants, not as a part of an explicit enhancement strategy, but as part of a wish to lead a "normal" life. For example, Jenny dreams of being able to cope with everyday challenges, just as she observes others doing. She says, "I just want to be able to sleep eight hours straight, be rested, do my homework, and live a normal life." Finding the right medication was a tiresome process, and Jenny had to test many different drugs before she was able to accept the level of negative side effects. Today she is content with the treatment: "I do the dishes, I wash my clothes, I go shopping, and I am well functioning!" Jenny pragmatically registers that the drugs enable her to do things that were previously unachievable, and even if getting there was a long way of experimentation, she is happy she continued the treatment.

In contrast to Jenny, who finally found the right medication and dosage, Kenny has decided to stop treatment. The initial excitement he experienced at the beginning of treatment unfortunately changed to disappointment end even anxiousness. His change in mood and general response to the drugs were too dramatic. Kenny explains:

KENNY: I had a really good effect from it. I have always struggled with my temper. I was irritable. But never after I got that [Ritalin]. My previously very short fuse was suddenly seven metres long and all pieces fell into place. Everything was quiet and calm and it was fantastic.

AUTHOR: What does it mean that all the pieces fell into place?

KENNY: Well, my head has always been a puzzle of two billion pieces, but now they suddenly fit each other.

AUTHOR: How did you experience that?

KENNY: Completely, wonderful calmness, and suddenly I understood things. I could do all the things I had never been able to do earlier. So that was nice. But after additionally six months, the negative side effects started, really really bad.

AUTHOR: What were they?

KENNY: Well, there were many. The psychosocial or what to call them. That was, I got totally careless, I couldn't laugh. I could watch the funniest movie, one I used to laugh my head off to, but I could not. I could not get angry either, I could not get sad. My mom died and everything and I could not even get sad. There were no emotions whatsoever. My son could come home from school and have had a really bad day and cry – I was totally indifferent. I mean cold as ice. I could not care less. If you saw a graph of it, it was just "biiiiis" – totally straight. No emotions at all, it was really scary, really. And then there were the more personal things, impotence, and then you are god damn not much of a man. That is not nice, I can tell you that. That was mostly … and then I lost a lot of weight. I did not sleep and I did not eat. It was like broken sleep all the time.

Kenny's story illustrates how balancing positive and negative effects of the treatment requires evaluation and determination. Generally, my interlocutors explain that taking medication eases the bodily and mental chaos connected to experiences of restlessness and racing thoughts. The effect of the drugs releases space for structuring thoughts and finding calmness, and many experience the positive effects of central nervous stimulants. However, complications with sleep, weight loss, vomiting, headaches, sexual problems, lowered mood, and tics are also reported as effects and the reason why a couple of the people I met during my fieldwork stopped treatment.

Asking my interlocutors about the experiences of taking medication, I learned that the practice of testing different drugs, judging their effect, and assessing levels and intervals of pill intake is an experimental process. It is a process in which individuals have new experiences. Every day and in all sorts of activities, drugs influence concentration, bring calmness, and make everyday activities manageable. Sometimes the drugs even influence the individual's perception and way of being in the world in staggering ways. Having always experienced restlessness and considered it as a part of one's being, the sudden calmness facilitated by drugs can be not only satisfying but also overwhelming. Being treated with central nervous stimulants is therefore not only a question of considering negative as well as positive effects, but also a question of experiencing oneself anew. Karen describes how she experienced taking her first tablet:

KAREN: I remember the first day, I was so excited and thought: it will probably not work. I got Ritalin to start with. Then I got home, and it was quiet, and I took the pill, and when 20–25 minutes had passed, not a damn thing had happened. The shitty drugs do not work! Bloody hell that is not okay! I got disappointed of course. And then some time passed. And all of a sudden, my head was just totally quiet. I promise you, it was quiet. And I was like, everything stood on end. So, I jumped over to the couch and sat down and waited till it was over, because that was just wrong! (Karen laughs)

AUTHOR: You had never tried that before?

KAREN: Never! So, I just sat there till it passed. Because I could not manoeuvre in it, it was wrong, it was crazy.

AUTHOR: What did you expect?

KAREN: Nothing, because what was I to expect? Nobody told me how others experience it. Nobody had explained what I should expect. (…) And it did not take long before, with this Ritalin, I got the feeling that I was a total wacko. Completely. I promise you it was wrong. Then it was quiet, then it was chaos, then it was quiet, then it was chaos. I mean it is the craziest thing I have ever gone through. Try to imagine that you have always been like that [restless and hyperactive] and then you get this drug and then someone pulls the rug out from under you, "swush", and you lay down there. And it is slippery, as you cannot even imagine. It is like being in an oil slick you cannot come up from and there are no edges to hold on to. You just float around. And you see it coming – that is actually the worst of it – but what? Why? You have no idea.

Karen's description is extraordinary in its intense character and emotional richness and not all my interlocutors give such a dramatic portrayal of their experiences with drugs. Karen's explanation demonstrates the experience of invasiveness on her being in the world. This way of being – a calm, non-chaotic state – seems strange when it is first encountered and experienced. How to relate to this way of being and how to assess if this is how it is supposed to be? Taking drugs may be a process of experimenting with new experiences. Karen is experiencing a profoundly different state of mind and being. All her life, her thoughts, bodily sensations, and actions have been chaotic and speeding, but taking drugs changes her condition dramatically, and consequently, it changes her relation with her children and her ability to be a mother. Karen tells me:

> The medicine has made it possible for me to have my life back. It has made it possible for me to enjoy my kids and be with them. I can help them and be there for them and give them everything I have in me.

Living a life in chaos had affected Karen's ability to take care of herself and her children, but the ADHD diagnosis and the subsequent treatment has helped her keep her thoughts straight – and, she tells me, it has been crucial in the path life has taken her.

A moral concern: becoming the person you want to be

Being diagnosed and testing different kinds of treatment produces doubts, hopes, and new practices. It directs the individual to a certain path, and promotes certain choices. The diagnosis brings about new considerations about how to live life and what to strive for, and everyday my interlocutors explore the possibilities of the diagnosis. Each day is an experiment in how life can be lived and while evaluating new treatment opportunities and challenges, each day potentially holds new ways of perceiving and being in the world.

Ann also describes how the medical treatment reduces her restlessness. These new experiences of calmness make her enjoy moments with her children more. The drugs give her "an inner calmness", and enable her to read bedtime stories to her children without having her "head speeding at 180 [km/h]". Being present in the moment and being patient with her children corresponds to the way Ann considers herself as a person and as a mother. However, the drugs also change her in less desirable ways and Ann continuously experiments with different types and dosages of medication in order to determine when side effects are acceptable, and when she is comfortable and able to recognize herself and her reactions. Ann explains:

> I would prefer to find the right medical treatment because I feel it helps me. But I do not want it to change my personality and make me different. I do not want my way of being and the way I act towards others to change. I have always liked that about myself. But I feel, I have noticed a tendency for me to be more egocentric, if you can say that. It is hard to put into words. But I have become a bit more introverted maybe. I feel I am more me when the drugs are effective and there are not too many

side effects. When it comes to treating myself nicely and taking care of myself, it is better with medication. But I sure need to get used to being on medication. A lot of things have been really good, because I feel like I am more patient with my kids and I do not go off as easily. And that, I feel, is more me. Sometimes [before the diagnosis and the treatment] I felt like it was not me going off, but it was something else doing it for me, and I was almost surprised by my reaction. And when it comes to that I think the medication has really helped me keeping calm and being the person, I would like to be.

Ann talks about experiences of being "more me" and being "the person I would like to be". Similarly, Karen speaks of drugs as enabling her to "give everything I have in me". A certain way of being "me" or a certain "self" is examined, strived for, and experimented with and the drugs become the facilitators of the experimental process. Changing moods, abilities, and perceptions, drugs work as "capsules of potentialities" (Trivelli, 2014, p. 159), creating prospects for another future and another way of being in the world. Sometimes the drugs change Ann so profoundly that she loses herself, while at other times the drugs help her to become the person she wants to be and who she recognizes as "being her". Karen and Ann, just like Kenny, are weighing up the consequences of taking drugs and they carefully experiment with new ways of being, rendered possible and experienced anew through the effect of medication. In this way, taking the medication is an experiment in hope and possibility as well as literally an experiment with experience in the assessment of how many, what kinds of, and at what intervals the medication must be taken in order to reveal the "real self" (Kramer, 1993). However, that real self is not a specific "self". The process of experimenting and striving does not have an exact goal or telos. Rather, this "self" is constantly experimented with in different contexts, with very different criteria. These experimental situations, in other words, are not a crossroads where the choice between left and right is clear-cut. Little changes in everyday life and changes in bodily sensations and reactions all become structuring for how Karen and Ann each assess themselves as a mother and as a good person.

Research examining the effect of Ritalin shows that the drug helps with self-management and regulates self-perceptions (Singh et al., 2010). Loe and Cuttino (2008), for example, examine how high school students diagnosed with ADHD strategically perform identity management in order to control their disordered body when striving to balance the experience of feeling true to the "authentic self "and managing the "ideal self" through negotiations of the "medical self". The students take medication to discipline themselves, as a kind of optimizing technology that gives them a sense of control. However, the medication may disturb the phenomenological experience of being true to oneself. The balancing act corresponds to Ann's experience of medication as both revealing and concealing what she recognizes as her real self. In this way, my interlocutors continuously evaluate the effects of medication. And while Ann and Karen continue taking medication despite unwanted side effects, Christian, another man I interviewed, decided to stop medical treatment because, as he says: "At some point I was so sick of medicine, I really just wanted to try being myself." Discussing the necessity of medication in order to perform academically or more generally in order to live up to the complex demands of the contemporary job market is of central importance and I will deal with the subject more thoroughly in Chapters 5 and 6. However, my interlocutors are not necessarily striving for an academic career. They experiment with different types of medication as part of a continuous striving for a manageable everyday life that enables them to do the dishes and read bedtime stories to their children without being distracted. What these people strive for is what most people call everyday life. Karen and Ann are experimenting with possibilities, new ways of experiencing and being in the world, and new ways of being a parent. The medication might be radical, but the assessment of the side effects and the evaluation of the drugs becomes part of a much bigger evaluation of the self, and a general process of becoming.

Concluding remarks

In this chapter, I have outlined different implications of being diagnosed with an ADHD diagnosis. The chapter demonstrates how a diagnosis and the following treatment produce narratives and new practices that all become part of a process of understanding oneself and of understanding life trajectories. The diagnosis is used as a part of a self-evaluative and self-constitutive project and it becomes a tool for structuring, evaluating, and experimenting with possibilities in life.

When people diagnosed with ADHD describe a chaotic mind and a chaotic life as their primary challenge and the diagnosis as the key to reordering their life, it illustrates aspects of what they hope and strive for. It also, however, tells us about the status of diagnoses and what normative demands the individual meets (and fails to live up to). It prompts us to ask the questions: How and why have psychiatric diagnoses become tools for self-understandings? And what does the need for a diagnosis tell us about our conceptions of how to manage adult life? Referencing Baumann (2007), Brinkmann (2016) argues that in a "liquid society", diagnoses metaphorically function "as anchors that somehow promise to solidify people's experiences of suffering" (p. 83). As an anchor in a liquid society, people diagnosed with ADHD use diagnosis as a solidifying, structuring element in a chaotic world. They struggle to meet expectations for leading an ordered life and pragmatically search for ways of anchoring their experiences of suffering. In that perspective, diagnoses become central actors in their evaluative projects of examining, experimenting with, and understanding themselves.

Acknowledgement

This chapter draws on work published in Nielsen, M. (2018). Structuring the self: Moral implications of getting an ADHD diagnosis. *Ethnos*, *83*(5), 892–908. Reprinted by permission of Taylor & Francis Ltd.

Note

1 For a thorough study of adults retrospectively rejecting their childhood diagnosis see Schwarz (2016).

References

Andersen, M. L. (2009). Former for ability: Hvilke Betydninger Tillægges en ADHD Diagnose i forhold til Selvforståelse, Intersubjektive og Institutionelle Positioner (PhD dissertation). Department of Sociology and Social Work, Aalborg Universitet, Aalborg, Denmark.

Baumann, Z. (2007). *Consuming life*. Cambridge, UK: Polity Press.

Brinkmann, S. (2014). Psychiatric diagnoses as semiotic mediators: The case of ADHD. *Nordic Psychology*, *66*(2), 121–134.

Brinkmann, S. (2016). *Diagnostic cultures: A cultural approach to the pathologization of modern life*. London: Routledge.

Conrad, P. (2007). *The medicalization of society: On the transformation of human conditions into treatable disorders*. Baltimore, MD: Johns Hopkins University Press.

Conrad, P., & Potter, D. (2000). From hyperactive children to ADHD adults: Observations on the expansion of medical categories. *Social Problems*, *47*, 559–582.

Goffman, E. (1963). *Stigma: Notes on the management of spoiled identity*. Princeton, NJ: Penguin Books.

Halleröd, S. L. H., Anckarsäter, H., Råstam, M., & Scherman, M. H. (2015). Experienced consequences of being diagnosed with ADHD as an adult: A qualitative study. *BMC Psychiatry*, *15*(1), 410–431.

Horwitz, A. V. (2002). *Creating mental illness*. Chicago, IL and London: University of Chicago Press.

Jutel, A. (2011). *Putting a name to it*. Baltimore, MD: John Hopkins University Press.

Kramer, P. D. (1993). *Listening to Prozac: A psychiatrist explores antidepressant drugs and the remaking of the self*. London: Fourth Estate.

Loe, M., & Cuttino, L. (2008). Grappling with the medicated self: The case of ADHD college students. *Symbolic Interaction*, *31*(3), 303–323.

Nielsen, M. (2018). Structuring the self: Moral implications of getting an ADHD diagnosis. *Ethnos*, *83*(5), 892–908.

Petersen, A., & Madsen, O. (2017). Depression: Diagnosis and suffering as process. *Nordic Psychology*, *69*(1), 19–32.

Rosenberg, C. E. (2002). The tyranny of diagnosis: Specific entities and individual experience. *Milbank Quarterly*, *80*(2), 237–260.

Schmitz M. F., Filippone, P., & Edelman, E. M. (2003). Social representations of attention deficit/hyperactivity disorder, 1988–1997. *Culture & Psychology*, *9*(4), 383–406.

Schwarz, A. (2016). *ADHD nation: The disorder. The drugs. The inside story*. London: Little, Brown Book Group.

Singh, I., Kendall, T., Taylor, C., Mears, A., Hollis, C., Batty, M., & Keenan, S. (2010). Young people's experience of ADHD and stimulant medication: A qualitative study for the NICE guideline. *Child and Adolescent Mental Health*, *15*(4), 186–192.

Timimi, S., & Leo, J. (2009). *Rethinking ADHD: From brain to culture*. Basingstoke, UK: Palgrave Macmillan.

Toner, M., O'Donoghue, T., & Houghton, S. (2006). Living in chaos and striving for control: How adults with attention deficit hyperactivity disorder deal with their disorder. *International Journal of Disability, Development and Education*, *53*(2), 247–261.

Trivelli, E. (2014). Depression, performativity and the conflicted body: An auto-ethnography of self-medication. *Subjectivity*, *7*(2), 151–170.

van der Geest, S., Whyte, S., & Hardon, A. (1996). The anthropology of pharmaceuticals: A biographical approach. *Annual Review of Anthropology*, *25*(1), 153–178.

Young, S., Bramham, J., Gray, K., & Rose, E. (2008). The experience of receiving a diagnosis and treatment of ADHD in adulthood: A qualitative study of clinically referred patients using interpretative phenomenological analysis. *Journal of Attention Disorder*, *11*(4), 493–503.

Chapter 5

Explaining and making use of an ADHD diagnosis

In the previous chapter, I illustrated how an ADHD diagnosis is not only used by doctors in order to categorize suffering and direct treatment, but that people diagnosed with ADHD also use the diagnosis as a resource for understanding themselves. Diagnoses are often criticized for being a means of social control in order to produce socially adjusted behaviour and diagnoses are said to produce new practices and identities (Comstock, 2011). In this chapter, I further examine how individuals diagnosed with ADHD relate to, engage with, and interpret the diagnosis as well as the explanations of it. I describe how my interlocutors, on the one hand, identify with ADHD as a specific way of being human and, on the other hand, distance themselves from ADHD by separating themselves from and disclaiming behaviour connected to ADHD. In different ways, I will argue that notions of ADHD as a brain disorder form the basis of both ways of relating to ADHD when adults are diagnosed with ADHD, in order for them to make use and sense of the diagnosis (Nielsen, 2017).

As part of my research, I interviewed Susan, who was diagnosed when she was 40 years old. I had been in touch with Susan on Facebook and noticed her profile picture: a cartoonish drawing of a man with an orchestra in the top of his head and a caption saying, "ADHD is like a symphony orchestra without a conductor." During the interview, I ask Susan what the profile picture refers to. "It explains what ADHD is," she replied, and further explains:

> Well, if we see it as a workplace, there is the doorkeeper in the back of the head who does not know how to close the doors so everything comes in … And then there are some confused employees in lack of a leader to tell them what to do so they are scuttling around like confused chickens. And then sometimes the frontal lobes are acting like the boss. So, all the knowledge is in the brain, but it is a long way sometimes because those neuro-things do not know their way so they are jumping around before they find their way, right. Well, I do not know. I do not know how to describe it.

All I know is that I find it harder to keep a sense of perspective and I get easily confused and stressed – easier than most people.

The picture was created by the Danish ADHD Association and I can see why Susan, a woman with a good sense of humour and a merry personality, has chosen the comical drawing as her profile picture. The picture illustrates Susan's identification with ADHD, her wish to be open about the fact that she is diagnosed with ADHD, and it represents an emerging tendency towards the destigmatization of psychiatric diagnoses. However, the picture also demonstrates how ADHD is commonly described and perceived: as a brain disorder. Susan's picture of ADHD as located in the brain points to a central theme in this chapter, namely the widespread neurobiological explanation for the condition. As I will show in this chapter, my interlocutors often refer to brain processes when explaining what ADHD is and how it is part of who they are, or when blaming the brain for making them act in certain ways. Since ADHD is often depicted as a neuroscientific fact, certain meanings are attributed to it, and certain actions flow from its consequences. During my fieldwork, I met various descriptions of how ADHD determines actions and ways of being, and even if some of the portrayals express complex ways of relating to ADHD, I have tried to outline two general positions. I have no intention of determining how to explain ADHD, rather my intention is to examine what kind of explanations prevail and how people make use of these explanations.

Dynamics between explanations and experiences

If you visit the official website www.sundhed.dk ("sundhed" means "health" in Danish), hosted by the Danish Regions and the Danish Ministry of Health), and search for "ADHD" you will find a short video explaining what causes the disorder. On a black background, the contour of a head with a fluorescent blue brain appears. We recognize the colours from pictures of brain scans and the video has a very "scientific" look to it. A voiceover explains (in Danish) that "attention deficit hyperactivity disorder (ADHD), is a frequent behavioural disorder caused by problems in the brain". The video zooms into the brain and we see from the graphics how neurotransmitters communicate information before the voiceover continues: "Some researchers state that ADHD is caused by a genetic error in particular neurotransmitters" and that "other theories point to the fact that poorly working nerve receptors that recognize dopamine cause ADHD". We are told about neurons, neurotransmitters, synapses, and receptors, and finally how symptoms of the condition are impulsivity, hyperactivity, and lack of ability to concentrate. The graphics guide us through the brain and the voiceover explains the mechanisms of all the different physiological processes in ADHD. In addition to the video, the website presents in text other possible factors behind ADHD such as environmental and hereditary components. But even if the voiceover in the video, just as the text describing environmental factors, presents different perspectives in understanding ADHD, the video has a different explanatory force than the text. The technique of imaging ADHD in this scientific, neuroimaging style, and the very concrete way of presenting the disorder makes a strong – and convincing – impression and leaves me asking: What are the implications of these explanations of ADHD on how we understand disorders, relate to them, and interpret symptoms? We know that a diagnosis may change people's self-perception, but how does the explanation of the diagnosis affect the way we think of ourselves and our difficulties? And may the explanations affect what options we imagine to have in terms of treatment and possibilities in life?

In order to address the above questions, I will outline some of philosopher Ian Hacking's ideas of how diagnoses are "making up people" (2007). In his book *Mad Travelers* (1998) Hacking examines fugue, a disorder first diagnosed and described in a publication in the late 1880s as a state of compulsively travelling and of obscured consciousness. After spreading across Europe, the diagnosis seemed to be forgotten, and today, the diagnosis no longer appears in the diagnostic manuals. So how is that? According to Hacking (1998), fugue is a "transient mental illness" (p. 13), defined by its character of appearing in a certain time and place and then eventually fading away. Illnesses come and go, diagnostic categories change, and social and cultural circumstances foster new illnesses. Transient mental illnesses therefore reflect what is considered pathological at a certain place and time. As a contemporary example, Hacking points to ADHD as a diagnostic category just recently emerged. We have known about fidgety children for a long time, but since ADHD is a relatively new diagnosis, both researchers and laypeople often question if it is a real disorder or a social construction. Hacking's interest, however, is not the question of whether disorders are genuine or not. Rather, he suggests that we understand the conditions under which certain mental illnesses thrive and that we examine the mechanisms of how diagnoses and individuals interact. Social and cultural contexts, or what Hacking (1998) calls "ecological niches" (p. 13), produce certain conceptions of the human and of the "normal" and "abnormal". Fugue, for example, emerged as a diagnosis in an age of tourism, when art and literature depicted adventurous journeys, but also in a time when the idea of the criminal vagrant scared people. These ideas about the wandering subject created specific conceptions of what healthy and unhealthy travelling entailed. Similarly, we may be able to identify particular conditions under which ADHD seems to grow. As noted by several researchers (see Chapter 2), various factors may account for the emergence of ADHD such as an increased focus on academic performance and self-management. Hacking (1998) argues that only by understanding the niches within which diagnoses occur is it possible to understand why diagnoses suddenly emerge and why some only shortly thereafter disappear again from the diagnostic manuals. Available descriptions in society offered by scientists, psychologists, therapists, the media, etc. make certain ways of being and experiencing possible, and the classifications into which we are put or put ourselves into, thus have a formative effect on how we understand ourselves.

As discussed in Chapter 3, Rose (2007) argues that in a time when we have become "neurochemical selves" who understand ourselves, speak about ourselves, and act upon ourselves and others as beings shaped by our biology, neuroscience plays a huge part in establishing what counts as explanations of a disorder (p. 118). Brain-scanning techniques, for example, are used by neuroscientists to investigate brain functions and potentially link hyperactive behaviour to abnormally functioning synapses (Comstock, 2011, p. 62). Within Hacking's theoretical framework, the proliferation of neuroscience into multiple disciplines establishes a niche in which human behaviour, preferences, and mental illnesses are explained in biological terms. Western societies today hold many specific perceptions of suffering, explanations for illnesses, and expectations of human capabilities, and within this niche, an ADHD diagnosis and its explanation offer a specific framework for understanding notions of being human. The emergence of ADHD as a diagnostic category and explanations of ADHD as caused by errors in neurotransmitters or poorly working nerve receptors establishes ADHD as something that can be pictured in a video, addressed with psychoactive drugs, and that can explain unwanted behaviour and sensations. New knowledge about ADHD brings about not only a label but also as Comstock (2011) puts it, "an identity that allows the subject to imagine and construct the self in new ways and in conformity with 'official' knowledge" (p. 57). By linking specific knowledge to a life trajectory, the diagnosis produces new meaningful identities and "kinds" of people.

In today's biomedical society investigating how people absorb and make use neurobiological knowledge is highly relevant. In his study on the role of mass media's depiction of mental illness on patients' perception of their condition, Dumit (2003) shows how people creatively make use of available knowledge or "received facts" (p. 39). We constantly fashion and refashion the way we think of ourselves based on translation of knowledge presented to us. However, as I write in Chapter 3, neurobiology does not exclusively determine how we think of ourselves as moral beings, even when diagnosed with what is conceived as a neurobiological disorder. Singh (2013) has analysed children diagnosed with ADHD and their discourses about self, brain, and behaviour.

Based on her research, Singh challenges what she calls the neurocentric idea that an articulation of a powerful brain necessarily leads to "a collapse of the self into the brain" (p. 817). Rather, Singh suggests, the children resist pressures to subjugate the self to the brain, and their discourses exhibit evidence of agency and responsibility despite having an ADHD diagnosis. On the one hand, the children strategically use the ADHD diagnosis as a resource in order to explain behaviour and morally disclaim responsibility, but on the other hand, they mobilize opportune behaviour based on certain conceptions of what ADHD is. Similarly, I will illustrate how my interlocutors make use of existing explanations of ADHD and how they creatively position themselves in relation to ADHD. I do not claim that people diagnosed with ADHD unambiguously subjugate the self to the brain, but I try to outline different positions and ways of relating to ADHD as a brain disorder.

Identifying with ADHD

In the beginning of this chapter, we met Susan, who downloaded a cartoon picture of an "ADHD brain" to use on her Facebook profile. Similarly, a great deal of ADHD merchandise is available online ranging from cups and stickers to t-shirts with "AD/HD" printed on the chest, referencing the logo of the rock band "AC/DC". The Danish ADHD Association sells jewellery such as a heart-shaped locket called the "wild ADHD heart" with "ADHD" engraved on the back of it, with an accompanying message describing the symbolic meaning of the locket: "Open it and show the world the true you. Close it again and be who you are. Carry the jewelry with pride." Goffman (1963) once described how people experiencing stigma make use of different strategies of stigma management by either trying to cover up the stigma or performing a voluntary disclosure (p. 125). Goffman suggests that people generally try to pass as "normal", not revealing their differentness. But as I describe in Chapter 4, concerns about discrimination when diagnosed with ADHD not only refer to the stigma attached to psychiatric diagnoses but also about the legitimacy of the diagnosis and convictions about who is rightfully diagnosed. Stigmatization is often related to not being acknowledged as someone with ADHD rather than of actually being labelled as someone with ADHD.

The industry of ADHD merchandise reflects an interesting phenomenon of people diagnosed with a psychiatric diagnosis, who take on the diagnosis, infuse it with pride, and use it as a resource. In her book on bipolar disorder, Martin (2007), who is diagnosed with bipolar disorder herself, writes about reclaiming the word "crazy", similar to the reclaiming of the word "gay" by homosexuals (p. xix). Insisting on owning one's diagnosis and taking pride in it indicates a new way of relating to psychiatric diagnoses. Rather than hiding the diagnosis, the use of ADHD merchandise illustrates a strategy of establishing ADHD as a legitimate identity by voluntarily disclosing it. ADHD is something to carry and hold with pride, as the description on the jewellery says. The diagnosis is not only accepted as a clinical explanation, it is also acted upon and employed as a way of expressing oneself. In that perspective, the clinical diagnosis is transferred into an identity marker to play with and relate to. How a diagnosis becomes a positive marker and undergoes a process of destigmatization can be explained in various ways. First, increased awareness about mental illness may have a positive effect on how people generally perceive people with mental health problems. Second, the explanations used for understanding mental illnesses may also have an impact on how people generally perceive concepts such as responsibility and potentiality. Research suggests that neurobiological explanations increasingly play a huge role in this matter.

Karen makes use of her ADHD diagnosis in order to understand herself and more specifically understanding the path life has taken and why she often felt misunderstood before being diagnosed. For Karen, receiving the diagnosis is about acknowledging and appreciating being in the world in a specific manner, existing under particular circumstances, and acting in certain ways. Karen identifies with ADHD as a way of being different, and the diagnosis has helped her understand how and why she is different. The consequences of not being diagnosed earlier have been severe, Karen's tells me, and she wishes she had been diagnosed when she was younger:

> I have always had it [ADHD], but I have never learned … no one ever showed consideration for me, I was never recognized as the person I am, which had the effect that I was not thriving. And it had the effect that I did not get to know myself and I did not use my resources appropriately.

Karen considers ADHD to be a fundamental part of her and she believes that the diagnosis has brought recognition and understanding of who she is, which earlier was never revealed or acknowledged. She has always been hyperactive "because hyperactivity keeps the brain awake", as she says, but she never learned how to use the hyperactivity constructively and was continuously reprimanded for her behaviour. Today, she is determined not to be ashamed of the person she is and to discover how to navigate in life, knowing that she is different from other people. Karen believes that because people with ADHD are different from "normal" people, they are made for another purpose:

> It is like we are all cars, but we are not made for the same purpose. A Ferrari drives extremely fast and someone is arriving as an old

Skoda. I mean hello, they are not made for the same thing. But they are vehicles. And then you have buses, but it is just a shame that I am not made for transporting passengers and that makes it difficult for others to understand.

Karen's explanation resembles many other descriptions of ADHD I came across during my research. Kelly describes herself as being like a plug with a grounding connection as opposed to a normal plug without a grounding connection: "In a normal power socket with only two holes, the plug with the grounding connection doesn't fit. I'm just made differently. You can say that I have more, I just do not have time to process it all." Similarly, Thomas draws a parallel between ADHD as another way of being human to different kinds of technical devices, describing himself as running another operating system than other people. I asked Thomas to elaborate on what he means by that, and he explained:

Well, let us say a computer uses Windows as its operating system. And then you run Windows, but it is not like … I just use another operating system! I control things differently. I mean … it is not a disadvantage, if you learn how to live with that. And you can. If you have the ability to take advantage of the impulsivity and the creativity you have because you are extra impulsive, you can create miracles, I think. But you have to live in this … well, I think if I had lived many, many years ago, I would prob-ably have been a good hunter and have been very well liked, but because I have to conform to this society, it does not comply with ADHD, so …

Thomas was diagnosed some years before I met him. As a young man, he tells me that he experimented with euphoriant drugs, "without knowing why I did it". Today, Thomas has started taking Ritalin, which enables him to keep a job and thereby provide for his two sons. The negative side effect, though, is a loss of creative energy. As he describes in the previous interview excerpt, he believes that the special skills he is equipped with are less valued today, but he acknowledges that he has to adapt. "People like me, you have to give us some pills, so you can be like a zombie and earn some money," Thomas says with a grin. The description of ADHD as another operating system was not new to me. On the online forums I followed as part of my research, a frequently shared picture depicted red flourishing, free floating, entangled organic lines on a black background with writing across the picture saying: "ADHD is not a system error, it is just another operating system." The picture gives associ-ations to electric voltage or human tissue studied through a microscope and the text teaches us that ADHD is not a human fault but just a different way of functioning. The idea that different ways of being, acting, and perceiving are caused by different "operating systems" or that the ADHD brain is "like an orchestra without a conductor", reflects a way of thinking about mental illness as caused by different biological designs of the human being. Both Karen, Kelly, and Thomas make use of these kinds of design references when describing people diagnosed with ADHD.

Both my interlocutors and also a large amount of literature on the subject explain human differences as biological variants – most of them based on a (neuro)biological understanding of ADHD. As an example, a genetic study of a particular Kenyan ethnic group has been used to explain ADHD as a product of evolutional adaptation (or the lack thereof) and why some particular receptor variants in the brain related to ADHD are an advantage for tribesmen living as nomads and a disadvantage for settlers (Eisenberg, Campbell, Gray, & Sorensen, 2008). The study was referenced in newspapers worldwide and used as an explanation of why some people do better under certain social circumstances and how natural selection has not adapted to the increasing urbanization of modern society. In their book on ADHD, Hinshaw and Scheffler (2014) suggest that a restless and exploratory character may have been a more valued trait in a hunter-gatherer culture when food was scarce. But in a world when academic performance is highly valued and sitting still for long periods of time is often necessary, this human trait has lost its significance. Though, the authors note, extremes of inattention and impulsivity may always have been problematic, if these characteristics affected hunting skills, for example, with a decrease in focus on the prey (p. 28). A similar perspective is presented by Thom Hartmann (1994), who associates ADHD with an evolutionary adaptation to the environment and the quality of prehistorical hunting skills. Within discussions about autism, the question of neurodiversity and autism as representing a different neurotype than the so-called "neurotypical human" is often raised (Silberman, 2015). Parallel to the position stating that ADHD is just another operating system or neurological variant, Silberman (2015) argues that autism is simply a naturally occurring cognitive variation that differs from the "normal" functioning brain and that rather than looking at autism, ADHD, and dyslexia as checklists of deficits and dysfunctions, these cognitive variants should be regarded as strengths that contribute with particular skills to the cultural and technological revolution (p. 16). Noticing, for example, that surprisingly many IT engineers in Silicon Valley have children diagnosed with autism, Silberman asks whether they represent a certain "tribe". Silberman's investigation of autism leads him to different "activists", one of them explaining why they refer to themselves as "autistic" instead of "people with autism". The young man explains: "We talk about left-handed people, not 'people with left-handedness' … It is only when someone has decided that the characteristic being referred to is nega-tive that suddenly people want to separate it from the person" (p. 441). These activists reject being constrained by a dominant conception of autism as a deficit and resist the subject positions following this stigmatizing conception (Davies, 2018, p. 38).

Similarly, my interlocutors emphasize that people with ADHD are different not sick, and Karen even describes how people with ADHD speak "ADHD'ish", following a different logic than others. ADHD is not defined as a disorder but rather a characteristic based on certain biological features. They are part of a biosociality (Rabinow, 1996) and share a biological citizenship (Rose & Novas, 2005) with others diagnosed with ADHD. In their research on adolescents' experience of having an ADHD diagnosis, Jones and Hesse (2018) elegantly describe the complexity of diagnosis as a means to control the individual as well as for the individual to experience a sense of control. They argue that

> by being conceived as a brain dysfunction, ADHD becomes an understanding that is applied not only to the difficulties of inattention, hyperactivity, and impulsivity, but also in some sense to the person as a whole, to their self-image, and to their identity.
>
> (p. 1)

According to the two authors, ADHD can be regarded as a "technoscientific identity" – an identity produced through the application of technologies as, for example, diagnoses. On the one hand, a technoscientific identity is inscribed upon individuals, who thereby are required to define themselves as lacking certain abilities (p. 2). On the other hand, however, a technoscientific identity can "work to increase a sense of control over experienced illness by applying biomedical information and characteristics directly to the person's sense of self and thereby encourage the person to *become* the classification" (p. 1). Within the framework offered by Hacking (2007), diagnosis makes certain ways of being and experiencing possible, and the classifications into which the individual is put or that they put themselves into, thus, has a formative effect on the individual's self-understanding. The person becomes the classification (Jones & Hesse, 2018). My interlocutors creatively engage with the diagnosis. They apply information about the diagnosis to their self-image and use the diagnosis as a mediator for understanding themselves as a technoscientific identity. However, they do not define themselves as "lacking certain abilities". Rather, they redefine ADHD as a particular way of being human, that they are somehow "made differently" or for another "purpose". Some researchers suggest that, in certain respects, "technoscientific identities [are] displacing illness identities" (Clarke, Mamo, Fosket, Fishman, & Shim, 2010, p. 26). Revealing the diagnosis and using the diagnosis and the explanations of it as something to carry with pride – and acknowledging different neuroversions of the human brain as performing diverse functions in society – opens up new ways of relating to the diagnosis. ADHD is much more than a disorder or a diagnosis. It is a specific way of managing (and failing to manage) based on certain neurological structures in the brain. Living in a society that favours certain behaviour over others might lead to unfulfilled expectations and experiences of failure and everyone I have interviewed emphasized that living with ADHD is challenging – even when knowing what causes the difficulties and how they are best managed. But my interlocutors oppose stigmatization and prepare for the challenges they meet. They identify with ADHD as a certain way of being human and insist on being accepted, understood, and helped with their difficulties.

Distancing from ADHD

While my interlocutors relate to ADHD as a category to identify with, they also sometimes distance themselves from ADHD. By distancing I do not refer to the act of rejecting or opposing the diagnosis, but I use the term to describe experiences of ADHD as something "other" that acts through them, something that takes control, and determines actions. Susan, for example, has difficulties controlling her temper, and, especially before she started taking Ritalin, she would often burst out with accusations. In the following, Susan explains how ADHD makes her react in ways she cannot recognize as hers:

> My common sense tells me that you do not yell into the head of a child or push it. That was definitely my ADHD. It was also my ADHD that made me react totally exaggerated if someone accidently touched me when I was on the bus. That is not me as a person because I am always happy and positive. I also wonder, how I could sometimes sit and talk to somebody, "la la la", and be happy, and then somebody just accidentally touched me, and then I was like "What the hell are you doing?" And then I suddenly became like, "I am really sorry." It just came out of nowhere. I mean, that is definitely my ADHD.

Susan's description of ADHD as acting through her and seizing her in ways she cannot avoid demonstrates a distancing between herself as a person and ADHD as an entity. ADHD is part of her, yet it is separate from her as a person. Susan identifies with ADHD and uses the diagnosis to understand her actions, but she also distances herself from it. Externalization is a common therapeutic technique for separating the problematic behaviour from the person in order to address the behaviour without blaming the person for it (White, 2007). The problem is the problem, so to speak, not the person. Brinkmann (2014) describes the process of transferring responsibility from the person to the entity of ADHD as an action of "disclaiming mediation" (p. 130). By converting a temperament or emotion into an object, or what Brinkmann refers to as "entification" (p. 128), the trait is separated from the person. Referencing a study of how ADHD is represented in the media (Schmitz, Filippone, & Edelman, 2003), Brinkmann (2014) describes the discursive process of explaining ADHD as a physical illness by depicting it though brain-imaging technology, and he connects the scientific brain discourse in the media to people's general perception of ADHD as an entity. According to Brinkmann, the element of understanding ADHD as being seized by a harmful agent is what constitutes the explanatory power of the diagnosis. Some kind of agent or entity inside the person has to account for the unwanted behaviour for the diagnosis to serve as an explanation. And so entification involves the necessary discursive creation of an agentic force inhabiting the individual. Similarly, in a study of adolescents' accounts of their ADHD-related behaviour, it is described how ADHD is positioned as an agent that overrules the individual's agency (Honkasilta, Vehmas, & Vehkakoski, 2016). Understanding troublesome conduct as caused by problems in the brain, the individual diagnosed with ADHD is perceived as a passive sufferer of a medical condition that therefore surpasses agency. In that perspective, ADHD offers a legitimate scapegoat, a factual, morally neutral, medical category that determines behaviour and emotions. If actions are determined by brain mechanisms, then the self is an actor "performing neuro-governed actions" (p. 254).

Kenny also makes a distinction between himself as a person and ADHD – or more specifically, between himself as a person and his brain. In this interview excerpt, he answers my question about what the diagnosis means to him:

> It makes me accept that this is how things are. It is not my fault. It gave me calmness to get the diagnosis because, ah, that is the explanation to why I have done as I have done and behaving bad. That is still comforting. Because if nothing was wrong with my brain or what to call it, then I would be the one having the problem, I mean Kenny the person and not my head. It cannot be an excuse, but it is an explanation. It is. To me.

Kenny has read a lot of literature about ADHD and knows about common explanations of it, but the description of ADHD as something "other" than him as a person is not only a theoretical explanation of brain mechanisms or a neurobiological discourse but also a very concrete, bodily experience of ADHD as acting through him (see also Chapter 6). He describes ADHD as tensions in his head, as electricity running though his brain, and he explains how the accumulation of energy in his body sometimes results in dramatic outbursts. He experiences a restlessness and bodily unease and he labels these experiences ADHD. Knowledge about synapses and neurotransmitters offers a language and an explanation that help interpret experiences in specific ways that connects these bodily sensations of electricity to brain mechanisms. In her auto-ethnographic study of depression, Trivelli (2014) writes, "when 'illness' takes over as the explanation of one's behaviour, unconscious processes, life circumstances and decision-making faculties turn into neurons, synapses or failed electric impulses. In this paradigm, one does not act. Illness does" (p. 157). Kenny's description of ADHD is similar: ADHD acts. It infiltrates his body and makes him react in inappropriate ways. However, distancing from the behaviour and bodily experience is not the same as rejecting responsibility or autonomy. Even if Kenny is distancing "Kenny the person" from "the head", he is emphasizing that he, Kenny, is the one who is responsible. Since he has identified his problems as ADHD, he is more aware of his reactions and how to cope with then, and he feels even more obliged to regain and not disclaim responsibility. Studies on experiences of ADHD and accounts of moral justification demonstrate a similar notion of responsibility. Asking young people about their moral responsibility, their responses revealed that medical explanations did not absolve them morally but on the contrary, they strived to be accepted as responsible agents (Honkasilta et al., 2016).

Rose and Abi-Rached (2013) argue that the influence of neuroscience does not imply a perception of personhood as brainhood. As they put it, "it's not that we are brains but that we have brains" (p. 22). The brain and its functions are brought into focus, but we do not incorporate the instrumentalist view that our brain solely dictates who we are as a person. The same is true for my interlocutors. Naturally, ADHD describes only certain aspects of the individual and is not sufficient to understand the whole person. However, researchers suggest that people tend to adapt neuroscientific knowledge into their self-perception if they have been provoked to consider their "brainhood" during a diagnostic process, that "[t]he brain may not intrude spontaneously in day-to-day consciousness, but rather becomes salient when something goes wrong" (O'Connor & Joffe, 2013, p. 263). In the event of a diagnosis, the functions of the brain, which are rarely the object of attention, become inescapably present. Paradoxically, while the so-called "normal" brain is considered passive and "lets the real self talk *through* it", the mentally ill brain "substitutes itself for the real self and speaks instead" (Dumit, 2003, p. 45). Normally we think of the brain as letting us be ourselves, but the opposite seems to be the case in terms of how we think of the brain in relation to mental illness. When Kenny experiences his thoughts as racing, and when he behaves contrary to his intentions, he understands this as a consequence of his brain. In this way, he draws on a neurobiological explanation of ADHD to interpret his bodily experiences and behaviour. However, Kenny's descriptions also demonstrate that brain mechanisms do not dictate who he is as a person, exactly because he is able to transform ADHD into an entity and knows what to distance himself from.

Within anthropological literature, analyses of spirit possession and rituals as healing teach us about conceptions of treatment and the power of naming experiences of suffering. In his study of chronic pain, Good (1994) describes how pain can provoke experiences of the body as an object, distinct from the acting self:

> The pain has agency. It is a demon, a monster lurking around, banging the insides of his body … At the same time, pain is a part of the subject, a dimension of the body, a part of the self.
>
> (p. 39)

While we normally consider the self as the author of our actions, that "we act in the world *through* our bodies" (p. 39), Good (1994) argues that the body becomes an object when it is in pain. Experiencing a force or an agent acting through you, it appears, is not exclusively connected to ADHD, but is a common human experience. Good (1994) refers to Lienhardt's study of the Dinkas, a people living in the southern part of Sudan, who are exposed to possession. According to Lienhardt, the Dinkas need to call out a name for the individual's suffering and create an image of the reason for suffering in a particular power in order to act on it:

> With the imagining of the grounds of suffering in a particular Power, the Dinka can grasp its nature intellectually in a way which satisfies them, and thus to some extent transcend and dominate it in this act of knowledge. With this knowledge, this separation of a subject and an object of experience, there arises for them also the possibility of creating a form of experience they desire, and of freeing themselves symbolically from what they must otherwise passively endure.
>
> (Lienhardt as cited in Good, 1994, p. 43)

In Good's (1994) analysis, medical treatment for chronic pain is like Dinka divination. By grasping the suffering as an agent and by calling out a name in the form of a diagnosis, an image of the pain is constructed in the body of the suffering person: "To name the origin of the pain is to seize power to alleviate it" (p. 45). For the Dinkas, as for Good and my interlocutors, the naming and the concept of suffering as an entity or an object is about grasping the experience in a way that satisfies us and corresponds to our cultural conception of the origin of suffering. While powers of possession legitimately explain suffering among the Dinkas, neurobiological explanations help Kenny, Susan, and others with similar experiences to understand their actions and bodily sensations and to act upon them. Experiences of tensions in the head, of losing control, and of bursting out are explainable and can even be pictured in an animated video as mechanisms functioning in specific autonomic ways. Only by making an entity of the suffering is it possible to distance oneself from it. And by distancing oneself from ADHD it is possible to manage the difficulties related to it.

Explanations of ADHD and expectations of treatment

When discussing with my interlocutors whether ADHD is a disorder or not, Jenny explains: "If you suffer from something that can be treated with drugs, then obviously you cannot say that it is part of your personality, because you do not treat personalities." According to Jenny, the answer is complicated. If ADHD is not a genuine disorder, psychiatry would not treat it. But as she elaborates later in the interview, ADHD and personality are intertwined: "Well, your personality is made in the brain, and if ADHD is implemented in the brain functions, then it is hard to separate." Jenny's answer exemplifies the complexity of how people diagnosed with ADHD relate to ADHD and, similarly, it illustrates the connection between the understanding of ADHD and decisions about its treatment.

During my research, I realized that a certain narrative about taking medication for ADHD is widespread: It was repeatedly described by the people I interviewed and by participants at online forums that medication prescribed for ADHD only work if you have ADHD. In his study on children diagnosed with ADHD, Rafalovich (2004) observes how abnormal brain activation, ADHD as a diagnosis, and the effect of medication is repeatedly connected. In order to confirm the legitimacy of the diagnosis, parents of children diagnosed with ADHD tend to link the effectiveness of stimulant medication to a validity of the explanation of their children's difficulties as brain problems (p. 165). Similarly, Schwarz (2016) notes that people diagnosed with ADHD often share the idea that a positive response to medication confirms the diagnosis. However, as Schwarz (2016) argues, central nervous stimulants invariably help the individual with ADHD to focus, just as it would help those without ADHD to focus. To claim that increased focus when taking medication confirms a diagnosis corresponds to a doctor saying: "Try these platform shoes, see if they make him taller" (p. 5). They obviously will. Taking medication that improves the ability to focus will inevitably help everyone focus better. But at the online forums and among several of my interlocutors, the effect of the medication is held to be the litmus test that determines whether you have ADHD or not, since the medication will have a relaxing effect if you have ADHD and a stimulating effect like amphetamine (which the medication is closely related to) if you have a normal functioning brain. Explanation and treatment mutually confirm one another: If ADHD is caused by a (dys)function of the brain, medication addressing that function is the solution; likewise, if the medication works as expected, the brain must be (dys)functioning in a specific way. Figuratively speaking, swallowing the pills means swallowing the meanings attached to them and vice versa. As John answers when I ask him why he started taking Ritalin, "I guess you follow the assumption that the drugs can do something to the brain, and well, then you have to try it out." Similarly, from his interviews with clinicians, Rafalovich (2004) argues that the hypothesis that ADHD is a neurobiological disorder is linked to the practice of prescribing drugs. As a kind of "reverse engineering" (p. 73) the available treatment comes to define the ailment it is treating, when the nature of ADHD is understood through the patient's response to medication. Comparable to earlier theories of hyperactivity, offered, for example, by Eisenberg, who claimed that effects of medication prove the diagnosis, contemporary theories of ADHD share the supposition that a positive effect of the medication proves the disorder (and its etiology).

In Chapter 2 I described how behaviour connected to what we call ADHD today has a long history of being considered a brain disorder that needs pharmaceutical treatment. Hyperactivity and inattention are, throughout the time when these types of behaviour have been considered medical cases, understood to emerge from different physical defects (Comstock, 2011). The explanatory model for understanding ADHD today has developed, but they still share some of the same features. Kleinman (1980) argues that ideas about the cause of illness are linked to ideas about treatment interventions. According to Kleinman, explanatory models "are held by patients and practitioners in all health care systems. They offer explanations of sickness and treatment to guide choices among available therapies and therapists and to cast personal land social meaning on the experiences of sickness" (p. 105). These models, determining what is clinically relevant, how the patient's symptoms are interpreted, and finally directing specific treatment, "are the main vehicle for the clinical construction of reality; they reveal the cultural specificity and historicity of socially produced clinical reality" (p. 110). Studying the rationales behind and consequences of different explanatory models therefore enables us to understand how both patients and healers experience and interpret illness. The models are anchored in particular cultural and social structures and arrangements, and being deeply immersed in the rules of different explanatory models, we often accept them without conscious reflection.

As noted by Fernando Vidal (2009), contemporary neurobiological explanations fit our Western conception of the human being as an autonomous self, and not only health professionals but also patients have endorsed the theories as a morally neutral way of explaining people's difficulties. In other parts of the world, however, different explanatory models resonate with people's conceptions of illnesses. The models differ in analytical power and level of abstraction, and while, for example, classical Chinese medicine considers most diseases as caused by "disharmony in the system of correspondences that extends from the cosmos to man" (Kleinman, 1980, p. 91), Western medicine often regards most diseases in terms of "the organ-specific lesions they produce" (p. 91). Understanding disease categories and etiologies differently therefore also leads to very different therapeutic actions. In another interesting anthropological study of different explanatory models, the anthropologist Ecks (2014) portrays how psychiatrists in India promote drugs as "mind food". Psychiatrists compare the act of taking drugs to the practice of eating in order to adjust the pharmaceutical treatment of mental disorders to the local conception of disorders as matters of digestion. Drawing on both local medicine's theories on balance as the prerequisite for health and digestion as the fundamental process in maintaining healthy, pharmaceuticals are presented as a " 'nutritional supplement' for the brain" (p. 5), for those who are in lack of a certain "mind food", just as some people need supplements for other conditions.

What we can learn from these cross-cultural comparisons of different explanatory models is how cultural narratives and explanations of illness and treatment are connected, and how patients' decisions about accepting the offered treatment often rely on whether the explanation and the treatment correspond. As Martin (2010) asserts, "Brain-centered understandings can lead to brain-centered interventions" (p. 379). This suggests that when you understand problems as being caused by deviances in the brain, you are more prone to both prescribing and taking medication that affects the brain. In the case of ADHD, medical treatment is effective and recommended by the authorities and most of my interlocutors have not only accepted taking medication but also experienced a positive effect from it. Sometimes, however, the neurobiological explanation, and the pharmaceutical treatment that follows it, fall short. John, who decided to accept taking medication because "it could do something to the brain", feels left alone with his problems after his visit to the psychiatrists, which only left him with a prescription for Ritalin. John explains:

It was just: "What kind of drugs should we prescribe? Do you think you need more or less? Should we increase or decrease the dosage?" I think they were really preoccupied with the drug thing. And: "We will try out some new drug if you experience problems with the current drug." But actually, I also needed to talk about some of the things I was fighting with at home.

Peter is also disappointed with the treatment he is offered by his psychiatrist. Not that he necessarily wants additional help besides the drugs but rather because they do not eliminate his problems. Peter had high hopes when he started treatment for ADHD, but he is not only surprised by the experimental process of finding the right type and dosage of the drugs, he is also disappointed with the uncertainty of psychiatry and biomedicine. Peter explains:

I cannot understand why science is not better than that. They have discovered how depression is caused by lack of serotonin in the brain, and how some substance in the brain, which I cannot remember, causes ADHD. So why have they not discovered what [drugs] to give you?

Peter is frustrated with science's inability to produce the exact substance his brain is missing. From reading about ADHD online, he expected the drugs to compensate for the deficiencies in his brain and thereby alleviate his problems. But even when he takes the drugs, he still experiences difficulties with overcoming everyday practices and keeping focus on tasks. The neurobiological explanation is not only descriptive and neutral, but it produces choices and hopes for treatment and generates certain expectations in its presentation of ADHD.

Neurobiological explanations of illnesses and the reduction of human experiences to brain mechanisms is widely criticized. Martin (2010) argues that neuroscience "claims to explain phenomena on one scale (those embodied for example in social relationships, places, practices and institutions that have a material existence outside the brain) by means of phenomena on another scale (those embodied in the brain)" (p. 369). In every explanatory endeavour, we tend to reduce complex phenomena of human social life, but the distinct feature of neuroscience's simplification lies in its insistence on the biological features of mental illnesses. Psychiatrist Thomas Fuchs (2012) has a similar concern and claims that neuroscientific explanations overshadow other explanations or simplify the dynamics of mental processes and therefore leave out other possibilities of treatment. Fuchs argues that as an organ of mediation of biology and social processes, the brain is embedded in interrelations between the social environment and the individual, and isolating mental disorders to brain structures only reveals one side of the coin. Nevertheless, as anthropologist Janis Jenkins (2010b) writes, "the pharmaceutical imaginary has come to pervade subjectivity as the cultural and existential ground in everyday life" (p. 17). As "pharmaceutical selves" we not only "orient ourselves towards drugs, but are produced and regulated by them" (Jenkins, 2010a, p. 4).

In the case of my interlocutors, pharmaceutical treatment is the primary treatment and only a few have been offered alternative help in the form of housing assistance, body therapy, psych education, and conversation therapy, and while such activities have been temporary, pharmaceutical treatment is considered lifelong. The conception that drugs can compensate for the impairment in the brain and that a certain response to drugs verifies the diagnosis leaves the individual in a position in which drug treatment seems to be the obvious choice. People are "participating in the world that psychopharmacology has opened up" (Martin, 2007, p. xix), and orient themselves towards the possibilities of a pharmaceutical treatment – even if the treatment occasionally fall short. On the one hand, my interlocutors welcome the pharmaceutical treatment, since it corresponds to the comprehension of ADHD as a brain disorder and not least help them manage their everyday life. But on the other hand, they experience various kinds of life problems, and while medication helps to reduce the unwanted effects of ADHD, complex problems sometimes require multifaceted solutions outside the realm of drug treatment.

Having or being ADHD?

During my fieldwork, whether I attended conferences, followed debates about ADHD, or interviewed people diagnosed with ADHD, the brain was continuously mentioned as the locus of the disorder. The message was that the ADHD brain works in certain ways, it prompts certain behaviours, and medical treatment can alleviate the unwanted symptoms. Moreover, the mantra, "you *are* not ADHD – you *have* ADHD" was repeatedly mentioned at every conference I attended, emphasizing that people diagnosed with ADHD are not their diagnosis and that ADHD is a disorder that needs treatment and ought to be recognized in the same way as diabetes or a broken leg. This biologization of mental illnesses (Rose & Abi-Rached, 2013) ranks ADHD alongside any somatic disease and explains ADHD as a matter of brain processes, just as diabetes is a matter of insulin production and a broken leg a bone fracture.

Brinkmann (2016) draws a parallel between the understanding of ADHD as an entity and "having" ADHD (p. 31). "Being" ADHD, on the other hand, is connected to an aspect of identity, and Brinkmann notes how the phrase "I am an ADHDer" is a common expression similar to saying "I am a footballer" (p. 31). In a study of adolescences' experiences of ADHD, it is suggested that these young individuals accept "having" ADHD, and that they seem to mobilize a psychomedical discourse in order to be recognized as a certain "kind of person" (Honkasilta et al., 2016). Being this certain "kind of person", however, is not the same as identifying as "being ADHD" (p. 254). The analysis contrasts another study of adolescents' experiences of ADHD (Krueger & Kendall, 2001), which concludes that the young people integrate their identity with the disorder, thinking that "they were their ADHD and their ADHD was them" (p. 64). To suffer from a condition, presumably located in the brain, confronts people with the dilemma (Dumit, 2003) of how to disavow the illness without disavowing oneself? The solution might be to create a new way of being human, which shares features with others diagnosed with ADHD.

What I came to learn from interviewing people diagnosed with ADHD was how ADHD is used in complex processes of understanding actions, sensations, and ways of being human. My interlocutors both identify with ADHD as a certain way of being human that needs to be recognized, and also distance themselves from ADHD by understanding it as an entity in itself that causes problems and suffering. Moreover, these different positions are not just discursive constructions or expressions of either being or having ADHD. The positions also represent bodily experiences of being caught by or directed by something "other" and ideas of being proudly part of a bio-social community of people sharing the same biology. ADHD needs to be treated since it causes various difficulties, but at the same time it needs to be acknowledged as a way of being a person. "You cannot cure ADHD, there's not something wrong with me. I'm just different. I'm not broken", as Kelly describes it. ADHD is not just a disorder; it is also a way of being human and the diagnosis is used as a mirror for interpreting humanness. Even if ADHD is considered a physical brain disorder and if the inattentive, impulsive, and hyperactive behaviour is a consequence of brain mechanisms, ADHD differs as a diagnosis from a broken leg, for example, because of the ways people diagnosed with ADHD relate to ADHD, act upon it, and use the diagnosis as a mediator for understanding themselves. Drawing a parallel between a broken leg or diabetes and ADHD often stems from an intention of recognizing mental illnesses equally with somatic disorders, which rightfully should be the case. However, few people suffering from a bone fracture or from diabetes would experience the condition as being connected to their sense of self – even if the condition affects your mood, daily routines, and future prospects. Moreover, while diabetes or bone fractures most likely are experienced as impairments with no obvious advantages, ADHD may cover a variety of features that sometimes complicate everyday endeavours and at other times (and maybe in other historical times) account for certain ways of talking, thinking, and behaving that are valued for being exactly what constitutes the person. ADHD is not only perceived as a collection of deficits, but additionally may also encompass potentialities.

New research reflects this complex and multifaceted approach to ADHD. In Denmark, for example, a new research project, headed by psychiatrist Per Hove Thomsen, studies how ADHD affects children's capabilities and quality of life. Part of the project further examines the positive aspects of ADHD, which include the possibility of children with ADHD managing certain situations better than other children. To focus on strengths and potentialities rather than deficiencies in ADHD can therefore help to reduce stigma and the general negative coverage of the diagnosis that may add to the existing barriers of thriving when struggling with ADHD. In her research on perceptions of psychiatric diagnoses, Martin (2000) describes how ADHD and bipolar disorder have undergone a revision in America, "from being simply dreaded liabilities, to being especially valuable assets that can potentially enhance one's life in the particular social and cultural world" (p. 512). Martin argues that ADHD appears as an asset in popular culture and in, for example, books for business entrepreneurs. Furthermore, authors such as Tom Hartmann and Edward Hallowell, as also mentioned in Chapter 2, have both contributed to the idea of people diagnosed with ADHD as being creative and having the ability to be a self-starter. Hallowell and Ratey (2005), also speak of ADHD as a collection of traits and a certain way of being in the world that can be transformed into assets. According to Martin (2000), traits considered as positive in psychiatric diagnoses reflect certain requested corporate proficiencies, and in a time when the labour market calls for competences such as fluency, flexibility, and adaptability, characteristics connected to ADHD may increasingly appear positive.

The tendency to value characteristics of ADHD and other psychiatric diagnoses seems sympathetic, and the effort to destigmatize people diagnosed with ADHD is commendable. Taking into consideration, however, that ADHD is determined on the basis of symptoms characterized as manifesting to a degree that is "inconsistent with developmental level and that negatively impacts directly on social and academic/occupational activities" (APA, 2013, p. 59), also makes one wonder what the status of diagnoses are if we start perceiving them as representing positive personal traits rather than a pathological condition. Whether the tendency contributes to a perspective that emphasizes the idea of "being" in preference to "having" ADHD, or identifying with as opposed to distancing from ADHD is uncertain. Nevertheless, the remaining task might still be to acknowledge and examine different – and sometimes contradictory – positions when interpreting how people diagnosed with ADHD relate to, make use of, and engage with the diagnosis in order to understand and explain themselves and their behaviour.

Concluding remarks

Researchers have pointed out that diagnoses are not only a tool for doctors to direct specific treatment, but that the individual who receives the diagnosis engages with it and uses it as a mediator for understanding themselves (Brinkmann, 2014; Jutel, 2011). As individuals, we are intertwined with the culture that we live in, and people diagnosed with ADHD are able to make use of the available technologies in order to better understand themselves and to help them navigate in a world full of challenges. Neurobiological explanations of mental illness and a general biologization of human behaviour and emotions shape how individuals think of their illness and difficulties in life (Rose & Abi-Rached, 2013). In this chapter, I have examined how ADHD is interpreted and related to by adults diagnosed with ADHD and how connections between knowledge, experiences, and technologies produce certain ways of understanding ADHD.

The analysis supports other studies pointing to the fact that an ADHD diagnosis not only stigmatizes or turns individuals into passive patients but also brings relief and leads to positive actions and an increased sense of responsibility (Halleröd, Anckarsäter, Råstam, & Scherman, 2015; Young, Bramham, Gray, & Rose, 2008). The way my interlocutors relate to ADHD does not entail a collapse of the self into the brain, even if they understand themselves and their difficulties in neurobiological terms. On the contrary, they creatively interpret what it means to be a human being with a specific neurologically structured brain. The chapter has shown that distancing from ADHD implies a separation of the self from the brain and an opportunity to act on ADHD, rather than being determined by the brain. Moreover, I illustrate how people can identify with ADHD as an alternative way of being human. I found elements of both positions of identifying with and distancing from ADHD in most of my interviews and my interlocutors did not hold one particular position, but rather they tend to switch between them when explaining different aspects of ADHD. Both positions involve the underlying premise that ADHD is located in the brain, but differ in their perspectives on the relation between the person and the brain.

Examining how people diagnosed with ADHD relate to ADHD and how explanations of ADHD affect decisions of treatment allows for a nuanced understanding of the dynamics between diagnostic explanations, self-understanding, and treatment. The chapter demonstrates that relating to ADHD involves complex and nuanced self-interpretations and actions, rather than a singular mode of interpreting the condition. However, the chapter also shows that identifying problems in neurobiological terms implies the acceptance of dealing with ADHD in a certain way, and additional or alternative strategies to drug treatment are often disregarded or less prioritized.

Acknowledgement

This chapter draws on work published in Nielsen, M. (2017). My ADHD and me: Identifying with and distancing from ADHD. *Nordic Psychology*, *69*(1), 33–46. Reprinted by permission of Taylor & Francis Ltd.

References

American Psychiatric Association (APA). (2013). *Diagnostic and statistical manual of mental disorders: DSM-5*. Washington, DC: American Psychiatric Association.
Brinkmann, S. (2014). Psychiatric diagnoses as semiotic mediators: The case of ADHD. *Nordic Psychology*, *66*(2), 121–134.
Brinkmann, S. (2016). *Diagnostic cultures: A cultural approach to the pathologization of modern life*. London: Routledge.
Clarke, A. E., Mamo, L. Fosket, J. R., Fishman, J. R., & Shim, J. K. (2010). *Biom edicalization: Technoscience, health, and illness in the U.S.* Durham, NC and London: Duke University Press.
Comstock, E. J. (2011). The end of drugging children: Toward the genealogy of the ADHD subject. *Journal of the History of the Behavioral Sciences*, *47*(1), 44–69.
Davies, A. (2018). Mapping the discourses of ADHD: The historical legacy. In M. Horton-Salway & A. Davies (Eds.), *The discourse of ADHD: Perspectives on attention deficit hyperactivity disorder* (pp. 27–68). Basingstoke, UK: Palgrave Macmillan.
Dumit, J. (2003). Is it me or my brain? Depression and neuroscientific facts. *Journal of Medical Humanities*, *24*(1/2), 35–47.
Ecks, S. (2014). *Eating drugs: Psychopharmaceutical pluralism in India*. New York and London: New York University Press.
Eisenberg, D., Campbell, B., Gray, P. B., & Sorensen, M. D. (2008). Dopamine receptor polymorphisms and body composition in undernourished pastoralists: An exploration of nutrition indices among nomadic and recently settled Ariaal men of northern Kenya. *BMC Evolutionary Biology*, *8*, 173.
Fuchs, T. (2012). Are mental illnesses diseases of the brain? In S. Choudhury & J. Slaby (Eds.), *Critical neuroscience: A handbook of the social and cultural contexts of neuroscience* (pp. 331–344). Chichester, UK: Wiley-Blackwell.
Goffman, E. (1963). *Stigma: Notes on the management of spoiled identity*. Englewood Cliffs, NJ: Penguin Books.
Good, B. (1994). *Medicine, rationality, and experience: An anthropological perspective*. Cambridge, UK: Cambridge University Press.
Hacking, I. (1998). *Mad travellers: Reflections on the reality of transient mental disorders*. Charlottesville: University of Virginia Press.

Hacking, I. (2007). Kinds of people: Moving targets. *Proceedings of the British Academy, 151*, 285–318.

Halleröd, S. L. H., Anckarsäter, H., Råstam, M., & Scherman, M. H. (2015). Experienced consequences of being diagnosed with ADHD as an adult: A qualitative study. *BMC Psychiatry, 15*(1), 410–431.

Hallowell, E. M., & Ratey, J. J. (2005). *Delivered from distraction: Getting the most out of life with attention deficit disorder.* New York, NY: Ballantine Books.

Hartmann, T. (1994). *Attention deficit disorder: A different perception.* New York, NY: Underwood Books.

Hinshaw, S. P., & Scheffler, R. M. (2014). *The ADHD explosion: Myths, money, and today's push for performance.* New York, NY: Oxford University Press.

Honkasilta, J., Vehmas, S., & Vehkakoski, T. (2016). Self-pathologizing, self-condemning, self-liberating: Youths' accounts of their ADHD-related behavior. *Social Science & Medicine, 150*, 248–255.

Jenkins, J. H. (2010a). Introduction. In J. H. Jenkins (Ed.), *Pharmaceutical self: The global shaping of experience in an age of psychopharmacology* (pp. 3–16). Santa Fe, NM: School for Advanced Seminar Series.

Jenkins, J. H. (2010b). Psychopharmaceutical self and imaginary in the social field of psychiatric treatment. In J. H. Jenkins (Ed.), *Pharmaceutical self: The global shaping of experience in and age of psychopharmacology* (pp. 17–40). Santa Fe, NM: School for Advanced Research.

Jones, S., & Hesse, M. (2018). Adolescents with ADHD: Experiences of having an ADHD diagnosis and negotiations of self-image and identity. *Journal of Attention Disorders, 22*(19), 92–102.

Jutel, A. (2011). *Putting a name to it.* Baltimore, MD: John Hopkins University Press.

Kleinman, A. (1980). *Patients and healers in the context of culture: An exploration of the borderland between anthropology, medicine and psychiatry.* Los Angeles: University of California Press.

Krueger, M., & Kendall, J. (2001). Descriptions of self: An exploratory study of adolescents with ADHD. *Journal of Child and Adolescent Psychiatric Nursing, 14*(2), 61–72.

Martin, E. (2000). Flexible survivors. *Cultural Values, 4(4)*, 512–517. Martin, E. (2007). *Bipolar expeditions: Mania and depression in American culture.* Oxford: Princeton University Press.

Martin, E. (2010). Self-making and the brain. *Subjectivity, 3*(4), 366–381.

Nielsen, M. (2017). My ADHD and me: Identifying with and distancing from ADHD. *Nordic Psychology, 69*(1), 33–46.

O'Connor, C., & Joffe, H. (2013). How has neuroscience affected lay understandings of personhood? A review of the evidence. *Public Understanding of Science, 22*(3), 254–268.

Rabinow, P. (1996). *Artificiality and enlightenment: From sociobiology to biosociality. Essays on the anthropology of reason.* Princeton, NJ: Princeton University Press.

Rafalovich, A. (2004). *Framing ADHD children: A critical examination of the history, discourse, and everyday experience of attention deficit/hyperactivity disorder.* Lanham, MD: Lexington Books.

Rose, N. (2007). *The politics of life itself: Biomedicine, power, and subjectivity in the twenty-first century.* Princeton, NJ: Princeton University Press.

Rose, N., & Abi-Rached, J. M. (2013). *Neuro: The new brain sciences and the management of the mind.* Princeton, NJ: Princeton University Press.

Rose, N., & Novas, C. (2005). Biological citizenship. In A. Ong & S. Collier (Eds.), *Global assemblages: Technology, politics and ethics as anthropological problems* (pp. 439–463). Malden, MA: Blackwell.

Schmitz M. F., Filippone, P., & Edelman, E. M. (2003). Social representations of attention deficit/hyperactivity disorder, 1988–1997. *Culture & Psychology, 9*(4), 383–406.

Schwarz, A. (2016). *ADHD nation: The disorder. The drugs. The inside story.* London: Little, Brown Book Group.

Silberman, S. (2015). *Neurotribes: The legacy of autism and the future of neurodiversity.* New York, NY: Avery.

Singh, I. (2013). Brain talk: Power and negotiation in children's discourse about self, brain and behavior. *Sociology of Health & Illness, 35*(6), 813–827.

Trivelli, E. (2014). Depression, performativity and the conflicted body: An auto-ethnography of self-medication. *Subjectivity, 7*(2), 151–170.

Vidal, F. (2009). Brainhood, anthropological figure of modernity. *History of the Human Sciences, 22*(1), 5–36.

White, M. (2007). *Maps of narrative practice.* New York, NY: W. W. Norton.

Young, S., Bramham, J., Gray, K., & Rose, E. (2008). The experience of receiving a diagnosis and treatment of ADHD in adulthood: A qualitative study of clinically referred patients using interpretative phenomenological analysis. *Journal of Attention Disorder, 11*(4), 493–503.

Chapter 6

ADHD as a temporal phenomenon

A headline in a Danish newspaper read: "They Don't Understand What I'm Saying, Because They Don't Think as Fast", citing a famous Danish model diagnosed with ADHD. The article was shared on an online forum and debated by the members of the group who commented on the model's hypothesis that people with ADHD think faster than other people and that differences in pace often creates misunderstandings. Opinions were divided on whether misunderstandings are due to the fact that most people think faster than they are able to communicate or whether they are due to the fact that people often tend to forget connecting links when telling a story. For example, one man proposed that

> the trick is to express yourself in a way so your thoughts can be perceived by others. Even if you have to put yourself in a slower tempo than your thoughts. And then lower your expectations to others' pace.

Many, however, declared themselves a fan of the hypothesis and agreed that people with ADHD have a certain "speediness" to their way of thinking.

I began this book by proposing that ADHD is a diagnosis of our time. Even if, as is suggested by some scholars, symptoms of what we characterize as ADHD today have been identified in children for a long time, the statistics of people diagnosed with ADHD bear witness to the fact that something inherent in contemporary society is at play. Something that directs our attention towards certain ways of being and acting, and that intensifies or increasingly renders symptoms of ADHD visible. In Chapter 2, I described how different disciplines explain ADHD and the emergence of the diagnostic category. Neither of these perspectives, however, address the experience of living with symptoms of ADHD or portray how everyday struggles with ADHD unfold within specific contexts and relations. In this chapter, I will contribute with an alternative perspective to our understanding of what ADHD is by examining ADHD as a specific way of temporally being in the world (Nielsen, 2017). During my fieldwork, I came to learn that time is central in experiences of ADHD and that timing, losing track of time, being on time, and tolerating the slow passing of time, was the subject of many concerns and frustrations among my interlocutors. Somehow, they always seem to be running out of time. They have difficulties finishing assignments on time, they show up late for appointments, and they sometimes need extra time before feeling comfortable in social settings. Time, however, is also often experienced as passing too slowly, as if the future cannot be awaited, and other people may seem slow, as the example in the beginning of this chapter depicts. Misunderstandings and experiences of being different, not being able to follow the expected track of time, therefore imbued the narratives about living with ADHD among my interlocutors. During interviews and spending time with my interlocutors I also felt confronted with the feeling of restlessness, misconnection, and misinterpretation, and I often experienced being at a different pace than the person I was sitting in front of. Restless movements sometimes overshadowed the interviews, my questions were interrupted whenever new thoughts struck the person I was in dialogue with, and our staccato conversations often took surprising directions.

The critique of psychiatric diagnoses is often, as I show in Chapter 3, that diagnoses locate the problem within the individual rather than in its surroundings. In this chapter, I try to nuance the perspective by showing how problems connected to ADHD exist in dynamics between the individual and their surroundings. In other words, I argue that ADHD is not only an individual phenomenon, but rather that ADHD appear in relations, clashes, interactions, and different contexts. I do so by exploring how to understand ADHD as a disruption in the experience of time and a state of desynchronization and arrhythmia. I illustrate how time is experienced as an intolerable burden and show how my interlocutors use different time-work strategies in order to cope with the obstacle of time. The perspective emphasizes the corporeal, embodied, and intersubjective elements of ADHD and calls for an acknowledgement of intercorporeality, that is, how bodies resonate with each other (Fuchs, 2014, p. 405). Hence, I suggest that symptoms described in the diagnostic criteria such as "avoids, dislikes, or is reluctant to engage in tasks that require sustained mental effort", "has difficulty organizing tasks and activities (e.g., difficulty managing sequential tasks; difficulty keeping materials and belongings in order; messy, disorganized work; has poor time management; fails to meet deadlines)", "is often 'on the go', acting as if 'driven by a motor'", and "blurts out an answer before a question has been completed" (APA, 2013) can be understood within a context of different, discordant rhythms, and desynchronization. I do not propose to explain whether the arrhythmia that I identify as part of the experience of ADHD is either cause or effect related to certain neurological processes; my aim is rather to offer a framework for understanding ADHD as an embodied and relational phenomenon. This perspective, I believe, can contribute to our understanding of ADHD not only as a neurobiological disorder or a diagnostic category that is "making up people", as Hacking (2007, p. 288) puts it, but also as a certain way of perceiving, acting, and being in the world.

Studying rhythms and experiences of time

Some scholars argue that, "Time is about coordination and rhythm, but it also involves material, emotional, moral, and political dimensions" (Shove, Trentman, & Wilk, 2009, p. 2). Time is at play in our interactions, our daily routines, and our engagement with the world around us. Spaces and technologies structure time and individuals experience, consume, endure, and manipulate time in different ways. Studying the relation between ADHD and experiences of time is not a new discipline, and several clinical experiments indicate that people diagnosed with ADHD have an impaired sense of time. Barkley and colleagues (Barkley, Koplowitz, Anderson, & McMurray, 1997; Barkley, Edwards, Laneri, Fletcher, & Metevia, 2001), for example, have tested children's ability to evaluate and reproduce temporal durations and conclude that children diagnosed with ADHD tend to under-reproduce certain time intervals (Barkley et al., 1997). From experiments measuring children's perception of time intervals, another study suggests that children diagnosed with ADHD tend to perceive time intervals as longer than others due "an internal clock that runs with a higher rate" (Walg, Oepen, & Prior, 2015, p. 2). According to the study, "brain structures affected by ADHD coincide with the presumptive neural correlates of temporal processing" (p. 1), which probably account for the children's alternative perception of time intervals. It is therefore also proposed, that "their impulsivity could arise from the fact that, from their subjective point of view, a rather long time interval has already passed" (p. 2). Similarly, in a study examining ADHD as a product of a diminished sense of rhythm, Gilden and Marusich (2009) suggest that people diagnosed with ADHD "have a rhythm cut-off that is faster in tempo than those without ADHD" (p. 265). By testing the ability of adults diagnosed with ADHD to synchronize and reproduce a metronome's rhythm, these researchers found that people diagnosed with ADHD start meandering or losing rhythm when the tempo is slowed down and therefore have greater difficulty than others in reproducing the rhythm within a certain temporal spectrum. From a clinical perspective, these studies illustrate the impairment of timely coordination and assessment in ADHD and can teach us important lessons about the condition. I, however, use a different approach when studying ADHD and temporal experiences. Taking my point of departure in rhythmanalysis, I examine ADHD as a rhythmic phenomenon by listening to stories of restlessness and understanding metaphorical descriptions of ADHD as mediators of experiences as well as by using my own bodily experiences of being with my interlocutors as data. Examining embodied experiences of ADHD through verbal communication has its limitations. However, employing a rhythmanalytical approach, I will demonstrate how verbal as well as bodily interactions offer access to embodied experiences and thereby help us understand ADHD as a certain way of being in the world.

In his book on rhythmanalysis, Lefebvre (2004) states that, "everywhere where there is interaction between a place, a time and an expenditure of energy, there is rhythm" (p. 25). I take this assertion as a fundamental point of departure in my study of the rhythms of bodies, thoughts, and interactions. Pointing to time as relative, Lefebvre describes rhythms as a measure: "A rhythm is slow or lively only in relation to other rhythms (often our own)" (p. 25) and "we each have our preferences and frequencies" (p. 20). Whether they are thought of in relation to societal rhythms of working hours, biological rhythms of sleep, or social rhythms of interactions, rhythms always exist in reference to something or someone. Our daily routines, habitual patterns, and ways of communicating all structure and are structured by certain temporal orientation. To study symptoms of inattention, hyperactivity, and impulsivity from a rhythmanalytical perspective therefore entails an investigation of ADHD as a relational phenomenon in reference to time. Here I draw on Fuchs (2013, 2014) and his theory of temporal experiences and states of desynchronization. When rhythms are not in accord, Lefebvre speaks of arrhythmia, and when differences in temporal experiences occur, Fuchs speaks of desynchronization. Both phenomena address the pathological, examine the moments of clashes, and point to processes of the body imposing itself. These perspectives therefore serve as the fundamental basis of my understanding ADHD as a rhythmic phenomenon and a desynchronized way of being in the world.

In analysing the interviews I conducted during my fieldwork, I was stunned by how my interlocutors used such a metaphorically rich language and the similarity with which they described their bodily experiences of ADHD. In searching for metaphors of experiences of ADHD, I found picturesque material of speed and energy accumulating. Metaphors of driving and racing were constantly used when describing ADHD, and I began to collect these examples to make an assemblage of accounts. Literature about metaphors points to their fundamental role in enabling us to conceptualize experiences. Metaphors both express experiences and structure our perception of the world and our way of navigating it (Lakoff & Johnson, 1994). In this perspective, our metaphorical descriptions and experiences are entangled, and experience and concept are one. Jackson (1983) states that, "[m]etaphor is not merely a figure of speech, drawing an analogy or playing on a resemblance for the sake of verbal effect" (p. 131), pointing to the idea that metaphors not only refer to something else or are used solely as comparisons or associations. Metaphors describe actual experience. Referring to Binswanger (1963), Jackson (1983) argues that when we use physical metaphors for emotional experiences, when, for example,

> disoriented individuals speak of the ground giving way beneath them, of being thrown, losing their footing, and of falling, these are not ... physical metaphors of mental states. Body and mind are effectively one, and what these images give evidence of is the actual experience of disoriented Being.
>
> (p. 9)

Jackson (1983) argues that a "metaphor reveals not the 'thisness of a that' but rather that 'this is that'" (p. 132). Thus, descriptions of, for example, a head speeding at 180 km/h and thoughts being a hodgepodge do not reveal the "thisness" of how ADHD is experienced. This is the actual experience of ADHD. The descriptions do not just serve as figures of speech; they are actual expressions of a speedy and chaotic being. On this basis, I use the metaphorical descriptions of ADHD as accounts of my interlocutors' actual experiences and ways being in the world.

While the people I interviewed during my fieldwork described feelings of being misunderstood, speeding thoughts, inner restlessness, and struggles with timing, I also often felt confronted with these feelings of restlessness during the interviews. The intuitive sense of being at a different pace therefore supported the metaphorical descriptions of ADHD I got from the interviews. I felt my own rhythm was challenged, and I used this information to support and elucidate what the people I interviewed were telling me about ADHD in terms of chaos and restlessness. According to Lefebvre (2004), to gain an understanding of rhythms, the rhythmanalyst needs to experience the rhythms through his or her own body, drawing "on his breathing, the circulation of his blood, the beatings of his heart and the delivery of his speech as landmarks" (p. 31). Lefebvre encourages researchers to call in their senses when studying rhythms to "arrive at the concrete through experience" (p. 31) and to pay attention to rhythms through concentration and by spending time in the field. He argues that "[t]o grasp a rhythm, it is necessary to have been grasped by it; one must let oneself go, give oneself over, abandon oneself in to its duration"

(p. 37). Inspired by Lefebvre, I used my own experience of being out of sync and sensing challenges to my own rhythm. Taking my own rhythm as a reference point in my research, using my body as a metronome, and trying to be grasped by or adapt to the rhythm of my interlocutors, I include my own experiences and notes from the interview settings to illustrate the feeling of desynchronization and of rhythms clashing.

The rhythms of the body

ADHD is about clashes, restlessness, and being unable to find inner calmness. That is how my interlocutors most commonly describe their experiences of ADHD and how they are most affected it. They explain that these experiences of restlessness manifest themselves as racing thoughts and a bodily craving for movement that overpowers other activities. John, for example, often experiences restlessness as something that builds up inside him, leaving him almost sick. When he sits by his computer, trying to focus on a task, or when he concentrates on reading a text, he feels an intolerable sensation of irritation and an urgent need to escape the situation. As he explains:

> I could get all sick from that inner restlessness that just wanted to get out or something. I had to act on it, I had to do something. It was like if you have to do something, but you do not know what. And it slowly builds up all the time, and gets worse and worse, and you do not know what you are supposed to do.

John's description of ADHD as a kind of restlessness reveals something central about the rhythm of the body. Something builds up inside and despite his intention of sitting still, concentrating on the task in front of him, he cannot do it. He has to do something, though he doesn't know what. John's experience of inner restlessness is almost unbearable, and he becomes desperate to ease the discomfort. He feels like he needs to act in order to endure the situation. Sometimes getting up and walking around can ease the restlessness, at other times John needs to lie down, close his eyes, and thereby escape the situation. John is constantly practising new methods for managing symptoms of ADHD and distracting himself (see Chapter 4).

The way John describes the feeling of inner restlessness resembles many other accounts of ADHD I collected during my fieldwork. Susan, for example, also portrays ADHD as a kind of restlessness. Especially when she is with her children and wants to provide an easy, calm space for them to be together in, she struggles with the feeling of restlessness. Being diagnosed and medically treated for ADHD, however, has made a difference for Susan in terms of being able to find inner calmness. In the following, Susan explains how medication changed her body – or the "tempo" of her body, as she puts it:

> I get an inner calmness. I guess that's the best way to describe it. For example, when reading bedtime stories to my kids, they are too big for that now, but when I did, it almost like … I did it, but it was not the nice experience that I wanted it to be – before I got the medication. Because my head was speeding 180 [km/h] while I was reading. I did not have the calmness to do what I was doing. I also tended to be really short-tempered and everything just shot out of my mouth and maybe sometimes inappropriately. The medication helps with that as well. It is a kind of general calmness in the body. I have so much more calmness in my body. But I have to get used to it; driving in a lower gear, if you can say it like that, and accept it. I find it quite hard realizing that my body feels drowsy in my world. But I guess that is just because I am in a normal tempo now. But compared with previous-me, this is drowsy to me and I have to accept that it is okay and do not feel guilty about not running around all the time.

The medication helps Susan to find "a normal tempo", and even if the current tempo seems drowsy to her, she appreciates the benefits. When taking central nervous stimulants, Susan manages to maintain the expected focus and establish the expected rhythm needed for dwelling in the moment of reading bedtime stories. A bodily sensation of calmness enables her to find interconnectedness with the situation and her children's need for attention. The setting demands focus, attention, and presence from Susan, and without the medication, her thoughts accelerate and she disconnects from the situation.

According to Lefebvre (2004), "the body consists of a bundle of rhythms, different but in tune" (p. 30). It is not only in music we find harmonies, but the body also "produces a garland of rhythms, one could say a bouquet" (p. 30). The rhythm of the body here refers to the beat of the heart, the repetition of breathing, and the circular element of rest, sleep, and work. Bodily functions rely on rhythms and produce rhythms when keeping the living organism alive. "Each segment of the body has a rhythm" and "these rhythms are in accord or discord with one another" (p. 47). The body is a polyrhythmic subject containing different rhythms that need to correspond or resonate in order to maintain health and rest in a state of what Lefebvre (2004) calls eurhythmia (p. 78). He continues:

> Rhythms unite with one another in the state of health, in normal (which is to say normed!) everydayness; when they are discordant, there is

suffering, a pathological state of which arrhythmia is generally, at the same time, symptom, cause and effect.

(p. 25)

If we think of the body as a polyrhythmic subject, an organism in need of harmonies and rhythmic resonance, we can see John's and Susan's experiences of restlessness as examples of bodily arrhythmia. Both experience disturbances in the body, as if something is not in accord, and both struggle to reestablish bodily comfort and well-being. It is not always possible to identify exactly the origin of arrhythmia, it rather appears as an all-encompassing restlessness. Sometimes, though, words burst out, inappropriately on certain occasions, as Susan explains, and the consequence of the inner restlessness becomes very obvious.

These kinds of unwanted outbursts are described by many diagnosed with ADHD. The arrhythmia often manifests itself as experiences of incongruence between mind and speech or body and mind, which sometimes cause misunderstandings in interactions with other people. Like Susan, Kenny describes his mouth as occasionally getting the better of him, especially if someone interrupts him or changes the subject in a conversation. He describes his speech as "like fire from another world', saying

> It is getting out of control and my mouth and brain are not connected any longer. It is running way, way too fast. It starts like if I am having carbonic acid in my arms and it has to get out.

While Susan uses Ritalin to provide a calmness in her body, Kenny makes use of another strategy. Since Ritalin had more negative than positive effects on him, he sticks to alcohol as a calming remedy. When his brain "runs amok", he drinks two bottles of wine, waits for the effect to kick in, only to throw it all up to avoid the hangovers, and then go to sleep. Kenny is well aware that the technique is unsustainable and usually he tries to shield himself from situations that may trigger his head to overload. But once in a while, he resorts to alcohol. Throughout the years, many relationships have ended due to Kenny's outbursts; and even more doors have taken a punch when he loses control. In a similar vein, Kelly explains how she is "too busy to sit down and understand what is going on" and reveals that she is sometimes ahead of herself, thinking faster than she speaks, especially before she started taking Ritalin. Kelly explains:

> I have been very flighty in my thoughts and in my construction of sentences, and earlier, it brought a lot of misunderstandings. I believe I have said a whole word or a full sentence, but I have not. A word such

as "not" is quite crucial in a sentence! If I have a sentence in my head, and I am about to say it, but I skip the essence while I keep on talking, it is not hard to see why people do not get it. So, in that perspective, there have been many misunderstandings and much frustration and I have been thinking: Why do people not understand what I just said? But I have not necessarily [said it].

Kelly and Kenny both have difficulties controlling their speech as they experience their mouths taking over, leaving rationality or specific words behind. There is a discrepancy between mind and mouth, and when distractions occur, these verbal stumbles happen. In the beginning of this chapter, I referred to the exchange of opinions concerning whether or not people diagnosed with ADHD think faster than others or if misunderstandings in communication are caused by a missing word or storyline. Kelly's description of her flighty thoughts resembles what is mentioned by some of the participants in the online discussion. Kelly feels she is "too busy", ahead of herself, she thinks so fast that she sometimes loses track. She explains the how it feels as if her head speeds too fast and her mind perceives too much:

> You do not have time to take everything in. You try to engage in 20 things, but you can only participate in one or two at a time. So, you have to cool down, pull over, and ask: How far did we get? What is our goal? And what can be saved for later?

From a rhythmanalytical perspective, we can understand the restlessness connected to ADHD and the feeling of speediness as a kind of rhythmic disharmony. Thoughts race too fast, blood runs too fast, and limbs move too much. And they do not always follow each other. The different rhythms of the different segments of the body are not in accord or do not resonate with each other and therefore create a state of arrhythmia. Falling asleep becomes difficult, concentrating on reading bedtime stories is almost impossible, and keeping track of words in a conversation is a struggle. The experience of inner restlessness draws attention to the physical body that is normally not present, and the bodily arrhythmia is experienced as disturbing and pathological. Philosopher Drew Leder (1990) describes how the body becomes the centre of attention in times of disturbance or illness. While the normal body is "essentially characterised by absence" (p. 1), in the sense that it "is rarely the thematic object of experience" (p. 1), the pathological body is characterized by an "absence of an absence" (p. 91), or what Leder calls a "dys-appearance" (p. 84). Lefebvre (2004) similarly describes arrhythmia as rhythms surging up and imposing themselves:

[N]ormally we only grasp the relations between rhythms, which interfere with them. However, they all have a distinct existence. Normally, none of them classifies itself; on the contrary in suffering, in confusion, a particular rhythm surges up and imposes itself: palpitation, breathlessness, pains in the place of satiety.

(p. 31)

When it feels to Kenny like carbonic acid is running though his body, his limbs call attention to them, revealing a disharmony. And when Susan realizes that her head is speeding at 180 km/h, her thoughts impose themselves, disturbing her ability to concentrate on reading and being in the moment with her children. Normally we ignore our body and presuppose that it "is just there". But experiences of a restless body and a speeding head interrupt intentions and expectations and reveal a particular discordance of rhythms and a "dysappearance" of the body.

When the world is at a different pace

Understanding ADHD as a phenomenon of bodily arrhythmia was my first analytical point in this chapter. By focusing on the intersubjective aspects of rhythms, my second argument points to ADHD as a desynchronization between the individual and their surroundings. My interlocutors continuously told me that they often show up late for appointments and that they find it difficult to manage time when working on a specific task. Judith, for example, explains:

It's just not there. The sense of time. It is now, now, now. It is about being in the present. That is how we are. I only just learned about time. Well, not watching the clock and seeing what time it is, but I mean sensing time and having an idea about how long things take. How long it takes to do grocery shopping and knowing when I will be back home again. Like getting a sense of it.

Diagnosed at the age of 45, Judith decided to become self-employed because she wanted to manage her own time and plan her tasks accordingly. In the previous interview excerpt, she illustrates why assessing time and managing time can be difficult: she genuinely experiences time as an incomprehensible phenomenon. From the psychiatric perspective presented by Barkley and his colleagues (1997; 2001), Judith's sense of time might be impaired. Judging time poorly creates misunderstandings and incongruences when making agreements and coordinating things with other people. However, my argument about ADHD as a certain temporal way of being in the world involves even more complex experiences of rhythmic confrontations. ADHD not only causes problems with time management in terms of handing in assignments in time or showing up on time for appointments. ADHD involves existential and phenomenological experiences of rhythmic disharmony.

In the following, Kenny describes how his experiences of bodily restlessness are often connected to certain situations. When he is expected to sit still and concentrate on a specific task, for example, a particular sensation in his body kicks in. Usually, Kenny tries to avoid situations he knows will generate these bodily experiences, but when obliged to participate, he knows how to manages these situations. Kenny explains:

KENNY: Mostly, I can feel the tensions here [he points at his head] and it is like … it is like trembling electricity through the brain "bizzzz". Those are the physical symptoms. And then I realize that I start shaking my legs [he is moving one of his legs restlessly up and down].

AUTHOR: What is up with that leg?

KENNY: Well, it is nothing now. But it is because the energy accumulates. And it has to come out somehow. When I go to a meeting, for example, where we have to sit on our butts and are being taught from the black board – then my legs start moving. I fiddle with something. It is like carbonic acid all over and that energy needs to be released. So, I will sit and jump a bit.

AUTHOR: So that is the valve?

KENNY: Yes, it is. It brings calmness.

During the interview, Kenny moves restlessly on the chair, waving his arms to underline his arguments, and he has a tic in his left eye. He speaks almost non-stop with great enthusiasm, gesticulating to emphasize his points. Kenny is a great storyteller and he expresses what several of my interlocutors recount as a speeding body that craves for movement. The experience of restlessness and the need for "calibrating" the body or letting the energy out when a structured time frame dictates how time is spent, was often described.

Difference in rhythm, however, not only happens when time is experienced as passing too slowly, it also exists between individuals. An excerpt from my field notes may exemplify how complex rhythmic confrontations often characterized my interviews and interactions with my interlocutors.

I am visiting Peter. We sit on his couch, it is morning, and we have a couple of hours to catch up from our last talk before I follow Peter to his psychiatrist. Peter describes how he still feels restless even though he has started taking drugs. Too many thoughts fill his head and he wants to discuss with the psychiatrist whether he should increase the dosage of medication. He slept badly last night. His girlfriend woke him up because he was kicking and moving toward her side of the bed. According to Peter, it is because he did not take his medication yesterday and never reached the deep sleep because of his restlessness. Peter describes his restlessness and how it affects his everyday life. My digital recorder lies on the table and records Peter's every word. But something – not caught by the digital recorder – illustrates Peter's restlessness just as well as his words. While we talk about his restlessness and his many thoughts, Peter is everywhere. He looks into his phone to check the alarm he sets in order to remember his medicine; he lights a cigarette with the lighter he has been fiddling with since we sat down; and he jiggles one of his legs throughout our conversation. Every time I ask a question, we somehow end up in a totally different place. I sense that I am getting confused from our staccato conversation, as we jump from subject to subject, and from all the activities happening during our conversation. Peter's restlessness fills the room. I get the feeling that we are speaking and thinking in different tempi and directions. Peter interrupts before I am done talking, not because he is impolite – he is one of the politest people I have interviewed – but because new thoughts keep striking him, independent of my questions and our conversation. I sense Peter's restlessness with much more than my hearing. It sneaks into my body. It crawls into my way of talking, as I have to stop my sentences half way through in order to adapt to our abrupt conversation. My concentration weakens as I follow Peter's eyes to his phone and to him lighting another cigarette. My breath almost shortens. I need to improvise to find common ground.

While Peter has difficulties finding inner calmness, the interview setting probably adds to his feeling of restlessness. I demand concentration on specific details and I guide our conversation following a certain structure, which I know is difficult for Peter. "I am way ahead. I am not even listening," Peter tells me when he describes how receiving details of an order from his boss or teacher is difficult, because he is already thinking about performing the task. When the conversation gets too slow, he starts meandering, like the test persons from the rhythmic experiments. I feel that Peter is already ahead of me too, losing focus on the present question.

In order to understand these clashes in rhythms, I turn to Fuchs (2014) and his theories on social synchronization. Fuchs is concerned with the phenomenology of mental illnesses and makes an interesting analytic comparison between different temporal orientations in states of mania and of depression. What characterizes mania, according to Fuchs, is "an acceleration and finally uncoupling of the individual from the world time" (p. 411). He continues:

The manic person is constantly ahead of himself, addicted to the seem-
ingly unlimited scope of possibilities. Interest in the present is always
distracted in favour of the next-to-come. The future cannot be awaited
and expected, but must be assailed and seized immediately.

(p. 411)

In some respects, Fuchs' description of mania resembles accounts of ADHD.
At a public seminar about ADHD, for example, a psychiatrist wittily suggested
that "for people with ADHD, it's about finding the brake pedal". Peter finds
it difficult to wait for his boss to deliver an instruction, and Kelly eagerly
stumbles upon the words. These experiences of impatience share features with
Fuchs' descriptions of constantly being ahead of oneself, of being distracted
by the forthcoming, and finally experiencing an "uncoupling" from the
surrounding world. Fuchs (2013) further emphasizes that our experience of
time is not a solipsistic phenomenon but it happens in reference to others.
There is an intersubjective element to experiences of time, as we engage with
and are ordinarily temporally synchronized with others (p. 81). The body is a
"resonance body" in which "interpersonal and other 'vibrations' constantly
reverberate" (Fuchs, 2014, p. 405). The body interacts with other bodies in
a continuous interplay of reciprocal understanding or intercorporeality.
Everyday contact with others therefore implies a "fine-tuning of emotional
and bodily communication and intercorporeal resonance" (p. 409) in order
to establish a feeling of being in accord with others. This fine-tuning or
social synchronization, however, can be challenged in various ways by either
"a retardation or acceleration of inner time in relation to external or social
processes" (Fuchs, 2013, p. 75), causing a state of desynchronization. We are
not always synchronized with our environment; we can be either "too late" or
"too early" (p. 81). Waiting, for example, imposes on us a slower time structure to which we may respond with patience or impatience.

If we return to the example of Peter and I, it seems like we are not following
the same rhythm, and that a kind of uncoupling takes place. Peter accelerates.
He is way ahead of me and becomes restless when I return to a previous
answer and ask him to elaborate. Our intercorporeal resonance and fine-
tuning are challenged by what I experience as Peter's acceleration and what he
probably experiences as me stretching out time. And we end up finding ourselves desynchronized. In a similar vein, Kenny and Susan's stories too offer
examples not only of inner arrhythmia but also of desynchronization. For
Kenny, attending a meeting is a confrontation with a specific time set. There is
probably an agenda for the meeting and a specific rhythm to the interaction.
Following the argument that people with ADHD have "an internal clock
that runs with a higher rate", as illustrated by experimental studies, we can

understand Kenny's impatience (Walg et al., 2015, p. 2). Kenny is confronted with another rhythm, another time than his own. The feeling of the energy accumulating in his body, as Kenny describes it, reflects the continuous accumulating time difference between his internal time and worldly time. Considering behaviour in terms of desynchronization, such as Kenny's impatience at the meeting, Peter's restlessness in the interview setting, or Susan's inability to concentrate on reading bedtime stories to her children while her thoughts are speeding, opens up a new way of understanding ADHD as a phenomenon that is not just located in the individual but that is also intersubjective or relative. The feeling of energy accumulating at Kenny's meeting, and Susan's conscious attention to her thoughts while reading bedtime stories, illustrate how confrontation with others creates a desynchronization that results in discomfort. Sometimes, the different rhythms of the body are not in accord with each other; at other times, the desynchronization happens between the individual and their surroundings. I differentiate between these two kinds of temporal differences, although they might happen concurrently. The mouth outpaces the brain when Kenny is interrupted; Susan's thoughts are racing, making the quiet situation with her children challenging; and Peter becomes restless and jumps from subject to subject when I interview him. All are examples of an inner state of arrhythmia in interactions with others or in specific contexts that demand a certain time structure, thereby resulting in desynchronization.

Social synchronization: trying to keep up but lagging behind

In an analysis of the importance of rhythm in social performance, King and De Rond (2011) suggest that "rhythmic synchronization is correlated with solidarity" (p. 76). Examining a boat race between legendary Oxford and Cambridge oarsmen, the authors describe how one team demonstrates a unity and creates a feeling of togetherness by moving together and finally winning the race. Only when a common rhythm is found is a social performance successful, and an experience of solidarity occurs. Although this makes sense in the case of rowing, it also makes sense in the broader context of being social, being in accord, and finding common ground.

My third point relates to a different aspect of time connected to ADHD. It is not about how ADHD is a different way of being but about the social consequences of this being. Many of my interlocutors remarked that the consequences of being different are dispiriting, and they often told me about feeling different, having difficulties with being social, and continuously experiencing social misunderstandings. In the following, Evelyn describes how she kept to herself before she was diagnosed and started taking Ritalin:

I have always been kind of ... back then ... I distanced myself ... and I have just been thinking: my brain is speeding so fast, and it actually ... it has always been like that with me. Because it was always racing. 20,000 thoughts. No one had any idea that it was racing like crazy in here. And I remember that, because it was also like that, when I was a kid. I could stay in my own world and those thoughts were just going around and round. I kept to myself. I was not open. But I was very observant, I remember that. And was thinking a lot of thoughts. I remember how I felt. And when I was looking at myself in the mirror I remember that inner ... I felt like ... I was restless inside and I felt like ... I don't know ...

Evelyn has a rich social life, takes dance classes, and enjoys being with others. Her weekly schedule is full, but once in a while she needs to cancel her plans and stay at home. "There are so many things I would like to do. But just the thought of it ... I completely burn [out]," Evelyn notes. The feeling of being different can lead to withdrawal from social settings, as can the feeling of having too many thoughts and too much restlessness, cause the need for social "timeout". In this way, the phenomenological being out of sync results (among other things) in a very concrete social desynchronization. What is normally felt as an indefinable difference, an abstract experience of a clash, sometimes leads to exclusion. Karen explains how her being different and needing to withdraw at times have severe consequences:

KAREN: I once read this piece that made me so extremely sad, and it still does. Someone was doing a presentation about ADHD, and when I saw the slides afterwards on the Internet, it said: It is not a question of whether you are excluded from sociality; it is a question of when you are. And I was so happy reading it first, but then I was so so sad.

AUTHOR: Why?

KAREN: Because it is true. I was being excluded, even though I still tried to be accepted and tried to keep at it, and tried to be like the others think you are supposed to be. And then it said it right there: it is not a question of whether but a question of when. And it is true, because you get no social training. You get a whole lot less because you have to withdraw. You cannot hold all that shit that is happening around you. So if you only get like a fourth of the social training compared to others, well then I am constantly 75 per cent behind. The result is, now that I am 45, I am supposed to manage that level of sociality, but I am not. There are a lot of basic things I am not able to.

Jensen (2017) uses the concept of chrononormativity from queer theory to analyse the general comprehension of autism as a development disorder and autistic individuals as being behind in terms of language and social development. In a queer context, chrononormativity is a description of heteronormativity applied to perceptions of time, and refers to the idea that queer persons are out of sync with society's expectations for people to follow a specific chronology in life (Freeman, 2010). In the context of expectations of social skills, people with autism often lag behind of what is expected. Similarly, Karen experiences that her social skills are weaker than is chrononormatively expected of adults. From a rhythmanalytical point of view, bodies are trained to follow the rhythms of calendars, institutional work hours, and interactions as part of a "dressage" of the body (Lefebvre, 2004, p. 48). There is a normative expectation of the individual, particularly from a certain stage in life, to rhythmically integrate into interactions without effort. Intercorporeal resonance happens in daily contact with others (Fuchs, 2013, p. 81), but withdrawal from sociality impedes the opportunity to establish and fine-tune synchronization with others. After years of socializing less than her peers, Karen cannot live up to the level of social skills expected from her as an adult in chrononormative terms and her desynchronization with others intensifies. The rhythmic synchronization has tough conditions, and it seems to be a vicious circle where the feeling of being different causes withdrawal from social settings, leading to a lack of social training. Every day, she tries to fit in. In order to avoid figurative "punches" from others, Karen tries to speak in a way that makes sense to others and to sit still on a chair when it is expected from her, as she describes in Chapter 1. Despite her good intentions and efforts to fit in, however, Karen still needs to withdraw sometimes and cannot catch up with others when it comes to fitting in.

By pointing out some of the social consequences of being out of sync, I am not suggesting that arrhythmia is a result of lack of social training. Rhythmic attunement and synchronization processes are complex phenomena that manifest themselves in both interactions and within the body. However, social interaction, as an art, requires rhythmic synchronization. At the centre of an interaction ritual, is what Collins (2004) describes as "the process in which participants develop a mutual focus of attention and become entrained in each other's present bodily micro-rhythms and emotions" (p. 47). Social activities are shaped by interaction rituals, and whether we participate in a boat race or in ordinary social interactions, a sense of connectedness and "successful collective performance" (King & De Rond, 2011, p. 583) depends on the entrainment of bodily rhythms. Karen, Evelyn, and my other interlocutors all struggle with rhythmic synchronization and thus with keeping up to the chrononormative expectations of their ability to socialize. The rhythmic disintegration and the feeling of difference are connected and shaped by each other, and the consequence might be social exclusion when failing to live up to others' expectations.

Developing time-work strategies

States of acceleration, restlessness, and experiences of uncoupling from the surroundings may cause some difficulties and lead to clashes and withdrawal from social settings. In order to adapt to the normative temporal regime, my interlocutors make use of various strategies – some involving different devices and some learned by carefully crafted practices. A number of tools are obviously used for structuring daily activities. Doctors' appointments, children's activities, and laundry-time slots are listed on white boards and scheduled in apps on smartphones in order to manage the frequency of activities and the allocation of time. The tools offer a visual overview of weekly activities, and alarms on the phone remind the user of the right time for taking the required medication. As mentioned in Chapter 4, structuring practices in new ways is often part of learning to manage symptoms of ADHD.

Similar to King and De Rond's (2011) analyses, sociologist Michael Flaherty (1999) argues that synchronicity constitutes interpersonal coordination and social order (p. 35). According to Flaherty, a central question in research when examining people's experiences of time is whether temporal experience is a product of "determinism", meaning situated factors beyond our control, or if temporal experience is the outcome of "self-determination", referring to the individual's arrangement of circumstances. We are not passively observing time. Rather, we engage with and experience variations in how time passes in different situations and due to different intentions. Therefore, Flaherty argues, we need to investigate the interplay between the self and the situation by looking into how people actively customize their experience of time when wanting to either stretch out time or make time pass faster. Participating in appointments structured around schedules, calendars, and seasons, we develop a correspondence between the flow of experience and the flow of the clock; and socially, we adapt into "the managed pulse of social interaction" (Flaherty, 2011, p. 47), as we tend to establish a rhythm to our activities. The concept of "time work", which Flaherty defines as "the intrapersonal and interpersonal effort directed toward provoking or preventing various temporal experiences" (p. 11), points to the activity of trying to influence how we experience time. "If our circumstances make for (or can be anticipated to make for) the perception that time is passing slowly, we 'act' in such a way that it seems to accelerate" (Flaherty, 2003, p. 22). Time work, therefore, not only refers to our social habitus and ability to internalize the temporal regimes imposed upon us, but also more specifically refers to the "agentic practices that are meant to control or customize temporal experience" (Flaherty, 2011, p. 149). Time work, in other words, is what people typically practice in order to "resist external sources of temporal constraint or structure" (p. 3). When circumstances are considered problematic, we strategically perform time work that alters our experience of the situation. We customize our temporal experiences in order to make time either pass quickly or slowly, by, for example, doodling in a notebook or thinking of places we would rather be (Flaherty, 2003, p. 22). Flaherty (2011) is concerned with the "doing" of time – whether consciously or unconsciously practised – and he argues that modifications of our own temporal experiences are "realized through the subtle and guarded practices" (p. 2).

During my fieldwork, I encountered various strategies among my interlocutors for conducting what Flaherty would call "time work". While the use of tools such as apps and white boards help organize time, other practices facilitate strategies of manipulating and customizing temporal experiences. When Kenny, for example, manages the bodily sensation of restlessness and the experience of time passing intolerably slowly by moving his legs up and down and fidgeting with a pencil, he performs a kind of time work. Similarly, Karen, sometimes unconsciously, walks around in her apartment to deal with the experience of things building up inside:

> Sometimes in the evening, when my head is overloaded, I get up and walk to the washing machine. I am not putting anything in it, I just walk out there and back again. I once asked myself: "Why on earth are you doing that? You have done it so many times with no purpose. You knew before going out there that the machine was empty and that you were not putting anything in it. But you walk out there anyway." Then I realized there is so much invisible noise in my head, which needs a little movement.

Karen laughs while telling the story. But she is also being serious. She needs these practices in order to endure situations when her head is overloaded. She needs the stimulation and release that it offers. Many people diagnosed with ADHD describe movement as a relieving practice, whether it be fidgeting with things, walking, or other kinds of bodily activity (Honkasilta, Vehmas, & Vehkakoski, 2016, p. 252). The opposite strategy to movement, however, may also suppress the unwanted restlessness. Paradoxically at first glance, but logically at further inspection, the use of ball blankets and ball vests points to a strategy for managing bodily restlessness. Having small balls sewn into them and being quite heavy, these blankets and vests stimulate as well as restrict the body and as a consequence, have a calming effect on the user. Kelly describes the use of her ball blanket as a strategy for being demarcated: "You are delimited. You are not floating. I don't know how to explain it. But otherwise, there's restlessness. So many thoughts and concerns." She coincidently learned how being held down by heavy weight had a relaxing effect on her.

After a rough period of eight days with no sleep due to bodily restlessness and racing thoughts, she collapsed on the couch – her head stuck in-between the cushions to avoid light and sound. Not until her boyfriend piled several duvets and blankets around her and tucked her in, his body weight on top of her, did she relax and fall asleep. After that experience, Kelly bought a ball blanket to simulate the same weight and sensation of being delimited.

Understanding temporal experiences as corporally embedded, I find these practices of managing the bodily symptoms of ADHD as techniques for experimenting with temporal experiences. Time work can be a means to resist temporal constraints, but time work may also, as the above examples illustrate, consist of techniques for enduring, responding to, and accommodating certain temporal structures. Anthropologist Mark Goodwin (2010) has analysed practices of body rocking and similar kinds of self-stimulation practices related to ADHD as moments of "becoming the moment" (p. 15). Goodwin claims that to become the moment means to "inhabit time without concern for the future (the main criterion of impulsivity), and thus to live differently in the present" (p. 15). Rituals of self-stimulation enable the body to become the moment – a body that "accrues time as a penalty in the form of under-stimulation, and that perceives this time as a burden" (p. 19). Body rocking, in this sense, holds a special relation to time because it consumes time. By performing body rocking the individual is immersed into a world they control, and time is made entirely its own, at least momentarily. In the same way that new technologies such as iPods and video games shelter us from the surrounding world, body rocking provides instant gratification and an affective method in which to "become the moment" (p. 50).

Goodwin's analysis points to a central aspect of time work. Becoming the moment means slowing down the acceleration of inner time, insisting on the present through movement or different kinds of body stimulation, and trying to synchronize with the surroundings by consuming time. When in a meeting, as Kenny describes, the absence of stimulation makes time unbearable, but moving his legs and letting the energy out is an act of inhabiting the body and connecting with the outside – and thereby to become the moment. Similarly, Karen experiences a desire for movement in order to accept sedentary situations. Knowing how others perceive her restless movements, however, she abstains from fidgeting with her hands and feet when she is not alone. She does her best to tolerate the unendurable stillness and to inhabit the present time. When alone, however, she restlessly moves around in her apartment, going back and forth to the washing machine. Consciously and unconsciously, my interlocutors experiment with time-work strategies, as they struggle to fit in, bear with their differentness, and to somehow rhythmically adapt to their surroundings. Opportunities for performing time work are dependent on the context and while movement, body rocking, and fidgeting may be suitable in some settings, these practices are not always appropriate or sufficient, and other kinds of techniques are needed.

As demonstrated throughout this chapter, synchronization is both a complex intercorporeal exercise, when individuals establish resonance through the fine-tuning of emotional and bodily communication and a practice of aligning with the temporal regimes of society. So, what is learned from understanding ADHD as a certain way of temporally being in the world? And how can the creative as well as pragmatic strategies used in everyday time work by people diagnosed with ADHD inform and develop treatment of ADHD? A growing literature focuses on the benefits of physical activities and mindfulness for children in general as well as specifically for children and adolescences diagnosed with ADHD (Månsson, Elmose, & Dalsgaard, 2017). Asking my interlocutors about experiences of practising mindfulness, however, often led to explanations of how they find the practice almost unbearable and exhausting in its insistence on doing nothing. Rather, Susan told me, she enjoys a body awareness programme she was offered by the municipality, because it teaches her new techniques for using her body. Whether mindfulness or other meditation practices reduce symptoms of ADHD is not to be determined here, but the potentiality of applying alternative practice when treating symptoms of ADHD is noteworthy. One specific study is particularly interesting when discussing alternative approaches to managing impatience, hyperactivity, and inattention: target-shooting sports as mental and bodily training have been shown to increase the ability to calm down and focus on specific tasks among children diagnosed with ADHD (Månsson et al., 2017). The study found that using breathing techniques and practising the ability to balance mind and body while shooting, children diagnosed with ADHD were able to enhance attention towards an object. As target shooting offers immediate feedback (you hit the bullseye or not), the exercise motivates children diagnosed with ADHD, who specifically struggle with awaiting the result of their efforts.

From an analytical perspective focusing on temporal experiences, the target-shooting research points to the benefits of "adapting the environment to provide a clear and concise structure, in regards to routines, time and space" (Månsson et al., 2017, p. 5). Structuring activities in ways that consider different challenges with temporal management and assist strategies for focusing on the here and now may be an alternative or supplement to pharmaceutical treatment. The complex art of "being in the moment", as Goodwin (2010) puts it, can counteract the acceleration of inner time and ultimately contribute to synchronization with the surroundings. "To enter into a society, a group or nationality is to accept values (that are taught) ... but also to bend oneself (to be bent) to its ways" (Lefebvre, 2004, p. 48). Whether it concerns breathing, movement or other bodily practices, people need to "learn to hold themselves" (p. 48), as part of the dressage of the body. The imperative of following the rhythm of society is unavoidable, however the potential of not only adapting to society, but also encouraging institutions to organize activities and learning environments that facilitates such rhythmic correspondence shows new ways for creating synchronization.

What is learned, then, from examining ADHD as a disorder of temporal impairment and as certain temporal way of being in the world, is how people diagnosed with ADHD use multiple techniques and creative strategies for managing symptoms of the condition. To think of these bodily techniques, people's choices of taking medication, or children's increased concentration and satisfaction with shooting games as practices of time work opens up for an alternative interpretation of individual deficiencies as well as agentic coping practices when adapting to norms for interaction. We experience time differently and therefore encounter different challenges in life related to adjusting and navigating in time. Some types of time-work practices may compensate for temporal discrepancies, but developing environments that facilitate concurrence and synchronism might also be part of eliminating experiences of temporal derailment.

Is society catching up on ADHD?

Throughout this chapter, I have proposed that ADHD can be understood as a desynchronized and speedy way of being in the world. People experiencing symptoms of ADHD may perceive the surroundings as too slow because of racing thoughts and a restless body. However, they often also find the outer world chaotic because their inner world is occupied with too many things.

One might think that a speedy being would be an advantage in a world where everything goes faster and faster. Rosa (2015) argues that modern society is continuously accelerating in all kinds of technological and social spheres. New computer models increase their processing speed every couple of months; the average time people spend sleeping and eating decreases; and changes of intimate partners and places of residence are also getting faster and faster (p. 63). The heightening of the tempo of life, "understood as an increase in episodes of action or experience per unit of time" (p. 78), results in an acceleration of actions and a stacking of actions such as multitasking, leading the individual to feel that they constantly lack time (p. 78). Initially this perspective seems to propose that synchronization between the person experiencing symptoms of ADHD and the surroundings would happen over time. If the time of a speedy individual is met by accelerating world time, then we might expect synchronization and the impatience and restlessness of the person might be neutralized as the world catches up. However, some researchers contradict this perspective, claiming that the complexity of modern society and changes of school and work conditions account for the increasing number of individuals who experience symptoms related to ADHD (Nielsen & Jørgensen, 2010; Timimi & Leo, 2009; see also Chapter 4). Acceleration is not necessarily productive. Indeed, it is often quite the opposite. Figuratively speaking, as a traffic jam is often the result of too many car drivers wanting to move too quickly at once, transforming speed into slowness (Edensor, 2010), so does over-stimulation and acceleration sometimes lead to distress and disablement.

When examining states of mental well-being as well as states of mental distress, Høgh-Olesen (2005) takes Rosa's argument further and asks: What are the personal consequences of the acceleration of Western society? According to Høgh-Olesen, each individual has an optimal level of stimulation, whereby the individual is neither bored from being understimulated nor stressed out from being overstimulated (p. 61). To answer his own question, Høgh-Olesen argues that the restless pulse of high-income industrialized societies causes an increased level of stimulation and so creates different kinds of mental deprivation, from anxiety to anorexia, for those who cannot cope with the bombardment of stimulation. In research on ADHD, it is widely acknowledged that impairment in the brain's reward system cause boredom and a strong reaction to environmental stimuli in people experiencing symptoms of ADHD (Gordon, Lewandowski, & Lovett, 2015). From this perspective, getting the right level of stimulation is a balancing act between under- and over-stimulation. DeGrandpre (1999) argues that ADHD is a product of a social environment with rapidly shifting media images and intensified demands of individuals being able to cope with ever-changing demands. ADHD, therefore is a result of an overstimulated populace plagued by too many sensory addictions, for which Ritalin becomes the equalizer. The question of synchronization, of being in accord with surroundings, therefore becomes a matter of accommodating to a society that keeps bombarding the individual with stimuli.

Modern society demands rhythmic synchronization in both social interactions and engagements with institutional, occupational, and domestic life. Lefebvre and Régulier (2004) speak of work as "the reference to which we try to refer everything else back" (p. 83). We organize the day according to our work. Our bodies are expected to adapt to the temporal regime of society and follow the rhythm of a seven-day week and eight-hour job. These disciplining practices, this dressage of the body in both social and institutional perspectives, require that individuals are capable of multitasking, managing time, and rhythmically adapting. Lefebvre (2004) contends that in military and sporting training, intervention through rhythm aims "to strengthen or re-establish eurhythmia" (p. 78), and Fuchs (2014) points to the benefits of resynchronizing therapy for people with depression in order "to give rhythm to everyday life" (p. 408). My interlocutors use various strategies for resynchronizing with the surrounding world, aligning with the temporal regimes of modern society, and overcoming feelings of restlessness. As described in this chapter, they make use of calendars and apps in order to remember appointments and take medication on time; they move the limbs in order to momentarily ease the experience of time being too slow; and they take medication as a strategy for creating calmness and strengthening the ability to concentrate and rest in the present moment.

To assume that an accelerating society and a speedy being fit perfectly together would be a consequence of taking both claims too literally. Symptoms of ADHD (and other disorders) do not ease when the pulse of society accelerates. On the contrary, demands of multitasking might trigger and aggravate feelings of restlessness and chaos. A bodily experience of racing thoughts or of restless limbs does not necessarily lead to a more productive everyday life (often the opposite) since the speediness often manifests itself as, for example, chaotic thinking, and jumping from task to task without finishing them, preventing productivity. An accelerating society only intensifies the experience of inner chaos and acceleration. What people diagnosed with ADHD need are strategies to find a valve, as Kenny describes it, or to put their thoughts in a slower tempo, as Susan explains, to find alternative strategies for resynchronizing not accelerating surroundings.

Concluding remarks

In this chapter, I have examined ADHD as a matter of difference in temporal experience and rhythm and I have argued that ADHD is manifested in an embodied experience of being out of sync. By using the metaphorical descriptions from my interviews with adults diagnosed with ADHD as portrayals of different ways of being in the world, I have illustrated how differences in perception of time, bodily restlessness, and the experience of speedy thoughts are connected, and how these can be understood within a framework of rhythm and desynchronization. Phenomenological research on rhythm and experience of time has guided my analysis and led me to conclude that ADHD can be understood as a rhythmic and desynchronized way of being in the world.

Following medical anthropologists such as Kleinman (1980), Good (1994), and Jenkins (2015), it is a central argument in this book that illness narratives are structured in cultural terms and that experiences of illness are always affected by available explanatory models and legitimate expressions of illness. So how can we examine experiences of ADHD without taking these explanations into account? My claim in this chapter is that even when acknowledging the entanglement of diagnosis and experience, and recognizing that experiences are informed by cultural narratives and available explanatory models of suffering, we may also as researchers address aspects of the different ways of experiencing that form our diagnostic categories and the social context in which these experiences unfold. I believe that a rhythmic perspective, as I have presented here, can offer an important contribution to the existing literature on and understanding of ADHD by examining it as a relational phenomenon and a certain way of perceiving, acting, and being in the world. My contribution is an attempt to investigate the phenomenology of the disorder in order to gain insight into the intersubjective elements and embodied experiences of ADHD. This does not mean that we should ignore the social structures and problems imposed by an accelerating society on people with symptoms related to ADHD. Rather, we should keep investigating how suffering can be understood and how different ways of being in the world unfold from multiple perspectives.

Acknowledgement

This chapter draws on work published in Nielsen, M. (2017). ADHD and temporality: A desynchronized way of being in the world. *Medical Anthropology*, *36*(3), 260–272. Reprinted by permission of Taylor & Francis Ltd.

References

American Psychiatric Association (APA). (2013). *Diagnostic and statistical manual of mental disorders: DSM-5*. Washington, DC: American Psychiatric Association.

Barkley, R. A., Edwards, G., Laneri, M., Fletcher, K., & Metevia, L. (2001). Executive functioning, temporal discounting, and sense of time in adolescents with attention deficit hyperactivity disorder (ADHD) and oppositional defiant disorder (ODD). *Journal of Abnormal Child Psychology*, *29*(6), 541–556.

Barkley, R. A., Koplowitz, S., Anderson, T., & McMurray, M. B. (1997). Sense of time in children with ADHD: Effects of duration, distraction, and stimulant medication. *Journal of the International Neuropsychological Society*, *3*, 359–369.

Binswanger, L. (1963). *Being in the world: Selected papers*. London: Souvenir Press.

Collins, R. (2004). *Interaction ritual chains*. Princeton, NJ: Princeton University Press.

DeGrandpre, R. (1999). *Ritalin nation: Rapid-fire culture and the transformation of human consciousness*. New York, NY: Norton.

Edensor, T. (2010): Introduction: Thinking about rhythm and space. In T. Edensor (Ed.), *Geographies of rhythm: Nature, place, mobilities and bodies* (pp. 1–20). London and New York, NY: Ashgate.

Flaherty, M. G. (1999). *A watched pot: How we experience time*. New York: New York University Press.

Flaherty, M. G. (2003). Time work: Customizing temporal experience. *Social Psychology Quarterly*, *66*(1), 17–33.

Flaherty, M. G. (2011). *The textures of time: Agency and temporal experience*. Philadelphia, PA: Temple University Press.

Freeman, E. (2010). *Time binds: Queer temporalities, queer histories*. Durham, NC and London: Duke University Press.

Fuchs, T. (2013). Temporality and psychopathology. *Phenomenology and the Cognitive Science*, *12*(1), 75–104.

Fuchs, T. (2014). Psychopathology of depression and mania: Symptoms, phenomena and syndromes. *Journal of Psychopathology*, *20*, 404–413.

Gilden, D. L., & Marusich, L. R. (2009). Contraction of time in attention-deficit hyperactivity disorder. *Neuropsychology*, *23*(2), 265–269.

Good, B. (1994). *Medicine, rationality, and experience: An anthropological perspective*. Cambridge, UK: Cambridge University Press.

Goodwin, M. (2010). On the other side of hyperactivity: An anthropology of ADHD (PhD dissertation). University of California, Berkeley.

Gordon, M., Lewandowski, L. J., & Lovett, B. J. (2015). Assessment and management of ADHD in educational and workplace settings in the context of ADA accommodations. In R. A. Barkley (Ed.), *Attention-deficit hyperactivity disorder: A handbook for diagnosis and treatment*. New York, NY and London: Guilford Press.

Hacking, I. (2007). Kinds of people: Moving targets. *Proceedings of the British Academy*, *151*, 285–318.

Honkasilta, J., Vehmas, S., & Vehkakoski, T. (2016). Self-pathologizing, self-condemning, self-liberating: Youths' Accounts of their ADHD-related behavior. *Social Science & Medicine (1982)*, *150*, 248–255.

Høgh-Olesen, H. (2005) Vestens puls. In A. D. Sørensen & H. J. Thomsen (Eds.), *Det Svære Liv: Om Lidelsen i den Moderne Kultur* (pp. 45–68). Aarhus, Denmark: Aarhus Universitetsforlag.

Jackson, M. (1983). Thinking through the body: An essay on understanding metaphor. *Social Analysis*, *14*, 127–149.

Jenkins, J. H. (2015). *Extraordinary conditions: Culture and experience in mental health*. Oakland: University of California Press.

Jensen, V. S. (2017). Performing autism through a layered account: Exploring the ambiguity of normative time and space. *Departures in Critical Qualitative Research*, *6*(1), 72–94.

King, A., & De Rond, M. (2011). Boat race: Rhythm and the possibility of collective performance. *British Journal of Sociology*, *62*(4), 565–585.

Kleinman, A. (1980). *Patients and healers in the context of culture: An exploration of the borderland between anthropology, medicine and psychiatry*. Los Angeles: University of California Press.

Lakoff, G., & Johnson, M. (1994). *Metaphors we live by*. Chicago, IL: University of Chicago Press.

Leder, D. (1990). *The absent body*. Chicago, IL: University of Chicago Press.

Lefebvre, H. (2004). *Rhythmanalysis: Space, time and everyday life*. London: Continuum.

Lefebvre, H., & Régulier, C. (2004). The rhythmanalytic project. In H. Lefebvre (Ed.), *Rhythmanalysis: Space, time and everyday life* (pp. 71–84). London and New York, NY: Continuum.

Månsson, A. G., Elmose, M., & Dalsgaard, S. (2017). The influence of participation in target-shooting sport for children with inattentive, hyperactive and impulsive symptoms: A controlled study of best practice. *BMC Psychiatry*, *17*(1), 1–6.

Nielsen, K., & Jørgensen, C. R. (2010). Patologisering af uro? In S. Brinkmann (Ed.), *Det Diagnosticerede Liv: Sygdom uden Grænser* (pp. 179–205). Aarhus, Denmark: Forlaget Klim.

Nielsen, M. (2017). ADHD and temporality: A desynchronized way of being in the world. *Medical Anthropology*, *36*(3), 260–272.

Rosa, H. (2015). *Social acceleration and the theory of modernity*. New York, NY and Chichester, UK: Columbia University Press.

Shove, E., Trentman, F., & Wilk, R. (2009) Introduction. In E. Shove, F. Trentman, & R. Wilk (Eds.), *Time, consumption and everyday life: Practice, materiality and culture* (pp. 1–11). Oxford and New York, NY: Berg.

Timimi, S., & Leo, J. (2009). *Rethinking ADHD: From brain to culture*. Basingstoke, UK: Palgrave Macmillan.

Walg, M., Oepen, J., & Prior, H. (2015). Adjustment of time perception in the range of seconds and milliseconds: The nature of time-processing alterations in children with ADHD. *Journal of Attention Disorders*, *19*(9), 755–763.

Chapter 7

Conclusion

This book is an examination of adults' experiences of ADHD. It studies explanations of ADHD, aspects of everyday life with ADHD, embodied experiences of ADHD, implications of being diagnosed with ADHD, and ways of relating to the diagnosis. Medical interventions as well as conditions of modern society affect perceptions of ADHD and the demarcation of who is considered within or outside the diagnostic category. Taking an anthropological approach, the book situates ADHD as a phenomenon and analyses experiences of ADHD within the context of our time, culture, and ways of understanding the human being.

As described in earlier chapters, research on ADHD often presents either neurobiological perspectives on ADHD, or explains ADHD as a consequence of environmental and societal developments. I have not positioned my research within any one of these explanations, but rather I have studied how these accounts influence individuals' experiences of ADHD. I have examined experiences of ADHD in relation to social relationships, family struggles, cultural explanations of suffering, and expectations of being human without understanding these experiences as simply products of social and cultural dynamics but rather in constant relation to them. Research on children's interaction with and understanding of the diagnosis is a growing field, and I hope that this book will contribute to an emerging field of sociological and anthropological research on adult ADHD.

In the following, I will first summarize some of the arguments and contributions of the book; second, I will point to avenues for future research on experiences of ADHD; and finally, I will discuss implications for practice based on the findings in the book.

Becoming someone with ADHD

Moral aspects of psychiatric diagnoses are often treated in examinations of diagnoses as distinguishing the normal from the abnormal, of stigmatizing effects of diagnoses, or of diagnoses as tools for social control – all perspectives dealing with social and cultural expectations of the individual. These insights illustrate how psychiatric diagnoses mark the transgression of moral boundaries and chart normative standards for behaviour and emotions (see Chapter 3). My analysis of the implications of getting an ADHD diagnosis examines another moral aspect of psychiatric diagnoses, as I focus on the individual's experiences of being diagnosed rather than assess the societal status of psychiatric diagnoses. In Chapter 4, I examine the formative process of getting an ADHD diagnosis and how individuals diagnosed with ADHD use the diagnosis as a part of a self-evaluative and self-constitutive project of becoming in the effort of structuring, evaluating, and experimenting with possibilities in a chaotic life. Following this line of reasoning, I argue that getting an ADHD diagnosis is a process in which existential questions are raised and everyday practices are scrutinized, evaluated, and often changed. Diagnoses offer new ways of being a person as well as new ways of relating to one's body, oneself, and one's environment. Experiences can be interpreted in a diagnostic context and pathological picture, and previous experiences are reinterpreted and verbalized within this framework. In a time and place when the diagnostic language dominates our way of understanding and making sense of suffering and when diagnoses offer legitimacy to people's experienced problems (see Chapter 3), people reach for diagnoses in order to cope with their difficulties.

The implications of getting an ADHD diagnosis are many. First and foremost, my interlocutors found the diagnosis a relief and welcomed it as an answer to the question of why they feel different. They understand the diagnosis as an explanation for their problems and use the diagnosis and the narrative connected to it as a framework for interpreting their life trajectory as well as a prognosis for their future. Rather than understanding their difficulties as a matter of moral derangement or some kind of flaw in character, the diagnosis reformulates these difficulties into a medical disorder. What were previously unspecified and abstract experiences in life are now transformed into a legitimate diagnosis. Moreover, resources following the diagnosis in terms of medication, guidelines, access to ADHD communities, and occasionally therapy or housekeeping assistance, help incorporate new routines and keep order in an everyday life that used to be chaotic. However, the diagnosis not only answers but also raises new questions and initiates moral deliberations about how to manage everyday difficulties. Taking medication, for example, involves reflections about when and how the individual feels comfortable and able to be the person they would like to be. Last but not least, the diagnosis often leads to concerns about stigmatization and feelings of ambivalence about now being labelled as "someone with ADHD". Other people's prejudices about who a person with ADHD is and what they are able or unable to do can form constricted frameworks for being in the world.

Explanatory models of ADHD

ADHD is portrayed and understood in multiple ways (see Chapter 2), and can be called, as Rafalovich (2004) puts it: "a socially negotiated phenomenon" (p. 178). Psychiatrists, social workers, teachers, and individuals living with the diagnosis may all have differing concepts of what ADHD is. Therefore, ADHD is a phenomenon that ranges from a medical category used for directing treatment to a category used in complex processes of understanding oneself. Historical accounts of ADHD demonstrate how inattentive behaviour and unruly children have been identified and treated within the medical arena throughout the last couple of centuries. Various physiological explanations of what causes the unwanted behaviour have been proposed, and while shifting medical regimes have suggested different explanations, the presumption that what we call ADHD today should be understood as a biological phenom-enon has a long history. Sociological research, on the contrary, points to societal development and medicalization processes that increasingly margin-alize and pathologize certain kinds of behaviour. Changes in school environ-ments, increased academic expectations, and a general request for continuous enhancement of the population produce new distinctions between individuals who either manage to navigate in and live up to these social circumstances or who fail in this endeavour. According to this perspective, ADHD therefore emerges as a category that identifies behaviour in need of treatment in order to adjust to society's requirements.

Looking at the dynamics between diagnostic categories and individual experiences, I study the process of applying ideas about ADHD on the individual's self-understanding. In Chapter 5, I examine the individual consequences of understanding ADHD within certain explanatory models and how biological accounts but also elements of sociological explanations of ADHD are integrated in ways of relating to the diagnosis. In Chapter 3, I discuss how neuroscientific models have gained ground in various fields of knowledge, both academic and public, and established certain criteria for how to think about and explain human behaviour. Neurobiological explanations of ADHD, for example, are often referred to when individuals diagnosed with ADHD discuss what the diagnosis is and how it influences their behav-iour and everyday life. When my interlocutors transform unwanted outbursts and unintended actions into an entity called ADHD that is acting through and seizing them in unavoidable ways, they make use of neurobiological understandings of mental illness as caused by brain mechanisms. Naming these experiences ADHD and explaining them this way, corresponds to our cultural conception of mental illness and enables a certain distancing from ADHD. However, while my interlocutors often explain ADHD as a consequence of brain processes, stating that the "ADHD brain" works in certain ways and prompts certain behaviour, these biological explanatory models are simultaneously linked to explanations that include more sociological aspects. When my interlocutors identify with ADHD as a particular way of "being human", based on neurological variations in the brain, which makes them struggle in our contemporary society, they also point to the narrowing concept of normality and the increasing demands for certain human capabilities. Using the diagnosis and the neurobiological explanations attached to it as something to carry with pride, new ways of relating to a psychiatric diagnosis appear and demand acknowledgement of people that may be "wired" differently performing different functions in society. In this perspective, ADHD is much more than an illness. It is a specific way of managing (and failing to manage), based on certain neurological structures in the brain, which is often at odds with cultural norms and expectations of behaviour in our accelerating, multitasking society.

ADHD as a relational phenomenon

Throughout the book, the dynamic relation between experiences and diagnostic category is examined, and I explore how experiences of mental illnesses are socially embedded. I argue that cultural narratives of illness inform experiences of ADHD and that experiences of ADHD are situated within relations, interactions, and in social contexts. Common to the perspectives is the exploration of ADHD as a relational phenomenon, which emphasizes that experiences of ADHD are intertwined with the desire to be a good parent, to be able to navigate in society, keep a job, maintain friendships, and be socially accepted. In Chapter 1, I introduced Karen, who told me how she had reached a point in life when her own strategies for managing no longer sufficed and that the diagnosis brought new resources to implement in her effort to navigate life. Karen and others diagnosed with ADHD that I have interviewed evaluate themselves in relation to their roles as a parent, friend, and employee. They orient themselves in the world based on expectations from themselves and others and their experiences of ADHD are shaped by and situated within their relation to others. Within our specific culture and place in time, certain ways of being in the world and certain ways of understanding and addressing individual problems and mental health issues are available, and experiences of ADHD exist within these particular circumstances. When life is chaotic, a diagnosis and treatment following the diagnosis may help structure everyday practices and thoughts and facilitate experiences of striving to meet one's own and others' expectations.

Examining ADHD as a relational phenomenon allows for alternative interpretations of ADHD. Even if the neurobiological explanation of the diagnosis renders various ways of relating to ADHD possible, the explanation might reduce understanding of how to live with ADHD and options for coping with the difficulties that it brings. In Chapter 5, I present a different perspective that emphasizes the intersubjective and intercorporeal aspects of ADHD and points to alternative techniques for managing symptoms of ADHD. The perspective illustrates how symptoms of ADHD appear in relations, clashes, interactions, and how different contexts intensify the symptoms. My interlocutors describe themselves as restless, unable to find inner calmness, and they explain how the feeling of restlessness manifests itself as racing thoughts and a craving for movement. These experiences of restlessness and feeling socially out of sync with others further provoke the experience of being different and misunderstood.

From a rhythmanalytical perspective, these embodied experiences of ADHD are examined as expressions of rhythmic disharmony and temporal desynchronization. In everyday activities, such as when attending meetings or reading bedtime stories to their children, my interlocutors are confronted with another expenditure of time than their own and the body imposes itself as restless or speedy. As social beings we constantly fine-tune bodily communication through intercorporeal resonance, but not everyone has the same preconditions for rhythmic integration. When time is experienced as a burden and rhythms are hard to follow, we find it difficult to socially synchronize with others or adapt to the situation we are in. The perspective therefore also opens up for an examination of the social implications of desynchronization and for a general discussion of the pace of modern society. In an accelerating society, when demands of multitasking and adaption to shifting milieus intensify, the risk of rhythmically losing track similarly increases. Individuals experiencing symptoms of ADHD therefore struggle to follow normative expectations of integrating into the rhythms of working hours and social interactions. Taking medication may be one way of managing symptoms of racing thoughts or bodily restlessness. However, as demonstrated in Chapter 5, various forms of creative bodily practices used in order to find relief and endure intolerable situations, also deserve careful attention and acknowledgement as ways of managing the symptoms of ADHD.

Avenues for future research

As with any research project, the analyses provided in this book not only answer questions regarding the experience of living with ADHD, they also ask new questions. Thus, the analytical findings presented lead to possible new areas of research. In this section, I will briefly propose future avenues for research that emerged from the analyses in the book and that deserve further academic attention.

During three years of doing fieldwork, I learned about the struggles of living with ADHD. Some of the people I interviewed were recently diagnosed with ADHD the first time I met them and were still exploring the implications of being diagnosed, while others had been diagnosed for many years. During an interview with Christian, discussing the time when he was diagnosed, he told me that he now thinks more pragmatically about the consequences of the diagnosis than he did during the years immediately following the diagnosis. When first diagnosed, he thought a lot about how to understand the diagnosis, what others thought about it, and how to deal with it. Now, four years later, he perceives the diagnosis as an integrated element in his life trajectory and circumstances. It is part of who he is. Maybe life could have turned out differently if he did not have these difficulties. And maybe even having these difficulties, he could have learned how to live with the problems without being diagnosed. But the diagnosis and the diagnostic process offered, as he put it, an opportunity for self-reflection. My interlocutors all reported that the ADHD diagnosis has helped them develop new perspectives and strategies to cope, even if they still struggle with everyday practices and in social relations. In evaluative processes of experimenting with different strategies for how to live life, the diagnosis serves as an instrument for interpreting challenges and opportunities. But, as Christian says, the implications of being diagnosed may change over the years. Similarly, concerns in life, abilities to manage life, and life situations might all change. Since my fieldwork lasted only three years, studying the implications of being diagnosed over the long term has not been possible. But asking questions regarding the long-term effects of being diagnosed could contribute with valuable perspectives on individuals' experiences of living with ADHD. Will the diagnosis, for example, become insufficient for understanding and managing new difficulties in life if the individual's life circumstances change? Will a diagnosis be inadequate and maybe even withdrawn if the individual develops strategies for coping with his or her difficulties in such a degree that symptoms of ADHD disappear? Research suggests that children sometimes outgrow symptoms of ADHD (Barkley, Murphy, & Fischer, 2008, p. 69; Jørgensen, 2014, p. 75). But can adults also develop in ways that render a diagnosis superfluous? And in that case, what are the implications on the individual's self-perception? Or what if the characteristics of the diagnosis change? For each new edition of the diagnostic manuals, diagnostic criteria change, which renders new ways of understanding suffering possible. What are the implications on individuals' identification with a diagnosis when diagnostic criteria change – if any? This book points to ADHD as being socially and culturally embedded, it emphasizes that experiences unfold in various contexts of interactions, and that the individual is constantly changing and formed by their relation with the world and others. An interesting avenue for future research could be to further study ADHD from a relational perspective and additionally examine how individuals diagnosed with ADHD relate to the diagnosis over the long term and through changing circumstances.

Another related theme that deserves further attention is the aspect of ADHD running in families. Research demonstrates that ADHD is a "highly heritable disorder" (Barkley et al., 2008, p. 384) and genetic examinations have provided insights into the heritability of ADHD, while anthropological research has contributed substantially to family aspects of ADHD. In an article introducing a special issue on "social contagion" and "contagious kinship connections", Meinert and Grøn (2019) examine why and how some disorders tend to run in certain families and kinship structures. As proposed by the authors, kin are often, yet not always, connected through genes. However, kin are also connected in the sense that they both touch each other's bodies through physical proximity and by sharing food, belongings, memories, homes, and places. They move and influence each other emotionally, psychologically, and existentially. The analysis could be seen to resemble the classic discussion of heredity and environment or nature and nurture, but the authors want to abolish this distinction and broaden the understanding of heredity by examining family relations, histories, illnesses, and misfortunes from a perspective inspired by hauntology. That is, a universal claim about the existence of a way of transmission. In research on adults diagnosed with ADHD, including my own, it often shows that parents are diagnosed after one or more of their children have been diagnosed with ADHD. Recognizing themselves in their children's behaviour inspires the parent to go through a diagnostic process as well. This indicates that symptoms of ADHD not only run in families due to biological connections but also because of certain behavioural patterns in families and a particular attention toward this kind of behaviour. Karen, for example, was diagnosed after her daughter's diagnosis. Karen explains:

> She [her daughter] is an exact copy of me, and I have really learned a lot about myself through her … When I see her, I see what other people see in me. I mean, if I feel like I am walking on a straight line, I am actually walking like this (Karen illustrates a staggering walk with her hands). I still feel like I am walking straight, but when I see her walking zigzag, I [think], "Oh that is what they mean!"

Karen has learned about ADHD through her daughter's diagnostic process, but she has also started to focus on the elements that constitute their family and their particular way of doing things. Jokingly she describes how visitors often feel abnormal in her family, because there is a certain family-way-of-being in her house. They behave in identical, uncommon ways. Similarly, Susan reflects upon her children copying her behaviour. Ever since Susan got the diagnosis, her outbursts have decreased and so have her children's.

Thinking about social contagion in relation to ADHD allows for examinations of how stories, habits, bodily features, and destinies are passed on from generation to generation. The perspective establishes a space for discussing how ADHD is transmitted within families through various connections as well as reflecting on how ADHD is enacted within families. How, for example, is a diagnosis received not only by the person diagnosed but also by the family? And what difference does it make if others in the family are already diagnosed – if any? Does age at the time of diagnosis matter? A couple of my interlocutors suspect that one of their parents might have ADHD as well, but none of them consider a diagnosis would make any difference for their parent, saying that "they have come to terms with how they are". The perspective also enables us to ask how families are affected by a diagnosis – how is awareness and care potentially altered or redirected toward new matters of concern? And what are the effects on a family's self-perception when one or more of the family members are diagnosed? Karen's description of the resemblance between herself and her daughter and the particular logic they share in her family illustrates how ADHD has become a constituent element in the family's perception of itself. When ADHD is understood as a certain way of being in the world (see Chapter 5), something determined by how your brain is neurobiologically "wired", this trait is possibly transmittable from one generation to the other. While this book has focused on the individual's experiences of ADHD in relation to the normative demands and societal structures they are surrounded by, it would be interesting to further study family dynamics and consequences in families in the event of one or more family members being diagnosed with ADHD.

Implications and recommendations for practice

Adults, to varying degrees, are responsible for their own actions and choices. If they see hyperactivity as a diagnosis that helps them understand themselves better and cope more effectively with what is a competitive and unforgiving world, then that is largely their prerogative. If they wish to take drugs to help "level the playing field", or give themselves an edge, that is also understandable.

(Smith, 2012, p. 184)

This quote by Smith reflects a pragmatic analysis of why adults are increasingly diagnosed with and treated for ADHD. Whether adults accept treatment for ADHD due to a perceived request for enhancement or because they find an ADHD diagnosis to be the key to an identity puzzle, both incentives make sense. Smith (2012) concludes, nevertheless, by stating that even if it is no surprise that adults resort to drug treatment, it is still sad that "we live in a society in which adults feel compelled to employ such measures" (p. 184).

I am certain that clinicians and other professionals working with ADHD are well aware of the complexity in adults' motivations for accepting a diagnosis and treatment of ADHD. Life-long experiences of failure, blame, misunderstandings, and confusion are to some extent explained and managed with a diagnosis in hand. And as Smiths (2012) notes, treatment of ADHD helps adults to cope more effectively. Sometimes, however, less transparent and maybe unintended consequences of being diagnosed surface. Acknowledging the effects of a diagnosis and reflecting over the consequences of being diagnosed with ADHD is therefore essential for both individuals with intentions of going through a diagnostic process and for health professionals. In this last part of the book, I will conclude by pointing to some recommendations for practice and ideas for reflections based on the analyses provided in the book.

First and foremost, I want to stress the importance of understanding the "life" of the diagnosis outside the clinic. Besides identifying, defining, and addressing symptoms, an ADHD diagnosis potentially alters self-perceptions, reflections over life trajectories and opportunities, and thoughts about personal responsibilities. The individual relates to the diagnosis in complex ways just as relatives, peers, and other people in the individual's surroundings do. Within this matrix of people relating and responding to the diagnosis, an ADHD diagnosis acts and is being acted upon. My interlocutors often experience that consultations with their psychiatrist mostly tackle questions of medication dosage and therefore they feel left alone with concerns about how to respond to others' perceptions of people with ADHD or maybe even their own prejudices about the diagnosis. Noting that receiving an ADHD diagnosis is not just a single event but a long process of understanding what the diagnosis entails is therefore important, and offering counselling that addresses the many questions emerging after being diagnosed is vital. I therefore encourage health professionals to continuously evaluate with their patients what role ADHD plays in their life, meaning both how symptoms of ADHD affect their everyday life and how the diagnosis is perceived and potentially prevents the individual from doing what they wish to do. Considerations about alternative means for managing symptoms and discussions about how to overcome experienced constraints, due to restricted conceptions of what people with ADHD are able to do, should also be addressed.

While the short- and long-term implications of being diagnosed with ADHD needs to be discussed, the positive effects of learning about the disorder and incorporating new techniques for managing symptoms of ADHD also require attention. What happens, for example, if the patient has learned to compensate enough for their difficulties to actually no longer meet the criteria for a diagnosis? When, if ever, is an ADHD diagnosis withdrawn? And in that case, what are the implications on the individual's perception of themselves, if the diagnosis helps them as a patient to understand and explain themselves and their difficulties? In a time when diagnoses are carriers of self-understandings and identity markers, and sometimes even associated with not only difficulties but also with special abilities, the role of the diagnosis is manifold. These issues of identity and interpretations of the self through a diagnostic logic need to be taken into consideration and discussed with the patient.

A related, but more radical issue concerns the question of whether the patient has the right to reject a diagnosis. Lotte Hvas (2015) provocatively insists on patients' right to deny a diagnosis in a society that, in her opinion, is on the verge of overdiagnosing individuals experiencing all sorts of problems. On the one hand, patients' motivation for walking into a psychiatrist's room is to get a professional evaluation and thereby potentially a diagnosis. On the other hand, the individual is not necessarily aware of the many implications of being diagnosed, and therefore discussing the effects of going through a diagnostic process and potentially living with a diagnosis is important.

Lastly, I encourage researchers as well as health professionals to include alternative interpretations of how to understand and discuss experiences of ADHD as well as management of difficulties related to ADHD. How will, for example, a rhythmanalytical perspective and a focus on rhythmic integration affect conversations in the clinical room about ADHD? According to Rasmussen and Meinert (2019), talking about ADHD as difficulties related to time and tempo offers a language that most people understand. Time is not a professional or technical concept linked to certain disciplines. Time is rather a common concept, and by talking about problems related to time rather than symptoms of ADHD, measures for managing difficulties are put on equal footing. Different explanatory models used for understanding ADHD provide different conversations about ADHD. Likewise, using alternative frameworks for interpreting certain difficulties potentially lead to new ways of understanding oneself as someone with ADHD.

With these final recommendations, I hope that the book will encourage researchers as well as health professionals to engage in discussions – preferably in dialogue with those being diagnosed – about living with symptoms of ADHD and the implications of being diagnosed.

References

Barkley, R. A., Murphy, K. R., & Fischer, M. (2008). *ADHD in adults: What the science says*. London: Guilford Press.

Hvas, L. (2015). Retten til at Være Rask i en Diagnosekultur. In S. Brinkmann & A. Petersen (Eds.), *Diagnoser: Perspektiver, Kritik og Diskussion* (pp. 319–340). Aarhus, Denmark: Klim.

Jørgensen, C. (2014). *ADHD: Bidrag til en Kritisk Psykologisk Forståelse*. København, Denmark: Hans Reitzel.

Meinert, L., & Grøn, L. (2019). It runs in the family: Exploring contagious kinship connections. *Ethnos* (forthcoming).

Rasmussen, G. V., & Meinert, L. (2019). ADHD – En Tidstypisk Tidsforstyrrelse? Tidsarbejde blandt Danske Familier der Lever med ADHD. *Tidsskrift for Forskning i Sygdom og Samfund* (forthcoming).

Rafalovich, A. (2004). *Framing ADHD children: A critical examination of the history, discourse, and everyday experience of attention deficit/hyperactivity disorder*. Lanham, MD: Lexington Books.

Smith, M. (2012). *Hyperactivity: The controversial history of ADHD*. London: Reaction Books.

Index